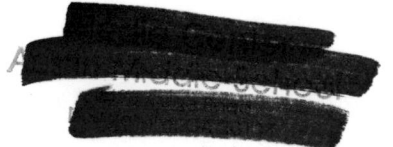

Great Medical Discoveries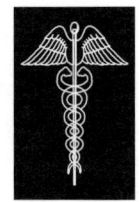

X-rays

by Craig E. Blohm

LUCENT BOOKS
An imprint of Thomson Gale, a part of The Thomson Corporation

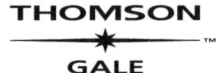

Detroit • New York • San Francisco • San Diego • New Haven, Conn. • Waterville, Maine • London • Munich

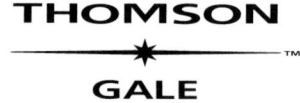

© 2005 by Lucent Books. Lucent Books is an imprint of The Gale Group, Inc., a division of Thomson Learning, Inc.

Lucent Books® and Thomson Learning™ are trademarks used herein under license.

For more information, contact
Lucent Books
27500 Drake Rd.
Farmington Hills, MI 48331-3535
Or you can visit our Internet site at http://www.gale.com

ALL RIGHTS RESERVED.
No part of this work covered by the copyright hereon may be reproduced or used in any form or by any means—graphic, electronic, or mechanical, including photocopying, recording, taping, Web distribution, or information storage retrieval systems—without the written permission of the publisher.

LIBRARY OF CONGRESS CATALOGING-IN-PUBLICATION DATA

Blohm, Craig E., 1948-
  X-rays / by Craig E. Blohm.
    p. cm. — (Great medical discoveries)
  Includes bibliographical references and index.
  ISBN 1-56006-933-3 (hard cover : alk. paper)
  1. Radiology, Medical—Juvenile literature. 2. X-rays—Juvenile literature. I. Title. II. Series.
  R895.B575 2005
  616.07'57—dc22   2004029042

Printed in the United States of America

CONTENTS

FOREWORD	4
INTRODUCTION A Tale of Two Presidents	7
CHAPTER ONE Diagnosing Disease	12
CHAPTER TWO Wilhelm Röntgen's "New Rays"	26
CHAPTER THREE X-rays in Medicine	41
CHAPTER FOUR Therapeutic Uses of X-rays	57
CHAPTER FIVE Improving Medical Imaging	71
CHAPTER SIX Images of the Future	86
NOTES	98
FOR FURTHER READING	102
WORKS CONSULTED	104
INDEX	108
PICTURE CREDITS	112
ABOUT THE AUTHOR	112

Foreword

Throughout history, people have struggled to understand and conquer the diseases and physical ailments that plague us. Once in a while, a discovery has changed the course of medicine and sometimes, the course of history itself. The stories of these discoveries have many elements in common—accidental findings, sudden insights, human dedication, and most of all, powerful results. Many illnesses that in the past were essentially a death warrant for their sufferers are today curable or even virtually extinct. And exciting new directions in medicine promise a future in which the building blocks of human life itself—the genes—may be manipulated and altered to restore health or to prevent disease from occurring in the first place.

It has been said that an insight is simply a rearrangement of already-known facts, and as often as not, these great medical discoveries have resulted partly from a reexamination of earlier efforts in light of new knowledge. Nineteenth-century monk Gregor Mendel experimented with pea plants for years, quietly unlocking the mysteries of genetics. However, the importance of his findings went unnoticed until three separate scientists, studying cell division with a newly improved invention called a microscope, rediscovered his work decades after his death. French doctor Jean-Antoine Villemin's experiments with rabbits proved that tuberculosis was contagious, but his conclusions were politely ignored by the medical community until another doctor, Robert Koch of Germany, discovered the exact culprit—the tubercle bacillus germ—years later.

Foreword

Accident, too, has played a part in some medical discoveries. Because the tuberculosis germ does not stain with dye as easily as other bacteria, Koch was able to see it only after he had let a treated slide sit far longer than he intended. An unwanted speck of mold led Englishman Alexander Fleming to recognize the bacteria-killing qualities of the penicillium fungi, ushering in the era of antibiotic "miracle drugs."

That researchers sometimes benefited from fortuitous accidents does not mean that they were bumbling amateurs who relied solely on luck. They were dedicated scientists whose work created the conditions under which such lucky events could occur; many sacrificed years of their lives to observation and experimentation. Sometimes the price they paid was higher. Rene Launnec, who invented the stethoscope to help him study the effects of tuberculosis, himself succumbed to the disease.

And humanity has benefited from these scientists' efforts. The formerly terrifying disease of smallpox has been eliminated from the face of the earth—the only case of the complete conquest of a once deadly disease. Tuberculosis, perhaps the oldest disease known to humans and certainly one of its most prolific killers, has been essentially wiped out in some parts of the world. Genetically engineered insulin is a godsend to countless diabetics who are allergic to the animal insulin that has traditionally been used to help them.

Despite such triumphs there are few unequivocal success stories in the history of great medical discoveries. New strains of tuberculosis are proving to be resistant to the antibiotics originally developed to treat them, raising the specter of a resurgence of the disease that has killed 2 billion people over the course of human history. But medical research continues on numerous fronts and will no doubt lead to still undreamed-of advancements in the future.

Each volume in the Great Medical Discoveries series tells the story of one great medical breakthrough—the first gropings for understanding, the pieces that came together and how, and the immediate and longer-term results. Part science and part social history, the series explains some of the key findings that have shaped modern medicine and relieved untold human suffering. Numerous primary and secondary source quotations enhance the text and bring to life all the drama of scientific discovery. Sidebars highlight personalities and convey personal stories. The series also discusses the future of each medical discovery—a future in which vaccines may guard against AIDS, gene therapy may eliminate cancer, and other as-yet-unimagined treatments may become commonplace.

Introduction

A Tale of Two Presidents

Friday, September 6, 1901, dawned clear and warm in Buffalo, New York, promising another hot day at the Pan American Exposition. A showcase of technological and cultural advances made by the nations of the Western Hemisphere, the exposition had opened on May 20 with a speech by U.S. vice president Theodore Roosevelt. As the fair entered its final months in the fall of 1901, President William McKinley was scheduled to deliver an address to the crowd. Among the thousands of people who flocked to the exposition for the president's address was a young man named Leon Czolgosz. He had come to Buffalo not to hear McKinley speak, however, but to kill him.

On Friday, the day after McKinley gave his speech, the president toured the fair and then stopped at the Temple of Music for a reception. A line of well-wishers formed outside to shake hands with the president, and at 4:00 P.M. the doors of the building were opened. As McKinley shook the hands of the people filing past, a man with a bandaged right hand approached the president. Before anyone could react, two shots echoed through the hall. Leon Czolgosz, with a handkerchief on his right hand to conceal a pistol, had shot the president. Czolgosz, an anarchist, would later tell authorities that he had done his duty. But there was still a chance McKinley could be saved.

McKinley was taken by ambulance to a hospital on the grounds of the exposition. Although one of Czolgosz's bullets had bounced harmlessly off one of McKinley's coat buttons, the other was embedded deep in the rotund president's body. In the hospital, McKinley was laid on a metal operating table and his wound was examined. Doctors decided to perform exploratory surgery to assess the extent of the damage the bullet had caused and to find and remove the bullet itself. As daylight waned, anesthesia was administered to the president and the operation started. The doctors repaired holes in McKinley's stomach, disinfected the area, and closed the wound in the abdomen. But they were unable to locate the bullet, which remained in the president's body.

That night McKinley was taken to a nearby house to recover from the surgery. For a week he remained stable and even improved somewhat. But by September 14, 1901, his condition had turned critical, and at 2:15 A.M. on that day, William McKinley died. The assassin's bullet remained somewhere in the president's body. In another room of the house sat an X-ray machine donated by Thomas Edison to assist in finding the bullet in the wounded president's body. The machine remained unused.

Eighty years later, on March 30, 1981, President Ronald Reagan was leaving the Washington Hilton Hotel in Washington, D.C., after delivering a speech to an audience of union workers. Walking with several aides and secret service agents, Reagan was about to enter his limousine when six pistol shots rang out. Suddenly the scene on T Street became one of chaos as several men were felled by bullets. Secret service agents and Washington, D.C., police officers lunged for the gunman, pinning him to the ground. The would-be assassin was John Hinckley Jr., a disturbed young man who thought he could win the attention of a movie star by shooting the president.

While the authorities were subduing Hinckley, Secret Service agent Jerry Parr quickly shoved President

A Tale of Two Presidents

Reagan into the waiting limousine. Feeling a sharp pain in his chest as Parr fell on top of him, Reagan thought that the weight of the agent had broken one of his ribs. When the president began coughing blood and experiencing difficulty breathing, the limousine sped to George Washington Medical Center. Once he was in the hospital's emergency room, Reagan began to collapse. At first, doctors had no idea what was wrong with the president. Had a broken rib punctured one of Reagan's lungs? Was he perhaps having a heart attack? The confusion ended when Reagan's shirt was removed, revealing a small hole under his left armpit. One of Hinckley's bullets had hit the president. And with no exit wound visible, the doctors knew that the bullet was still in Reagan's body.

At around 3:00 P.M., less than half an hour after he had entered the hospital, an X-ray was taken of the president's chest. The film clearly showed the bullet lodged behind Reagan's heart. Another X-ray was

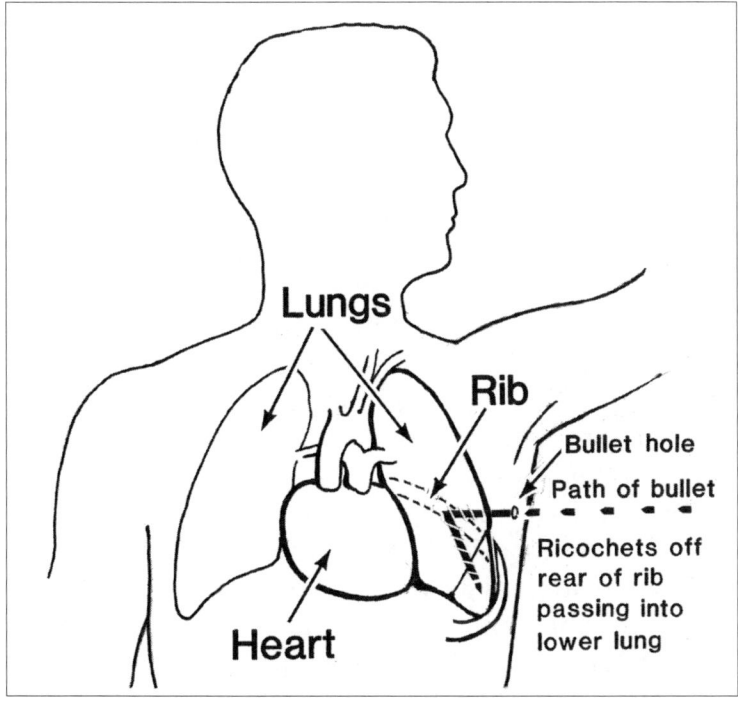

A diagram illustrates the path an assassin's bullet followed through the body of former president Ronald Reagan. X-rays helped doctors locate the bullet in time to save Reagan's life.

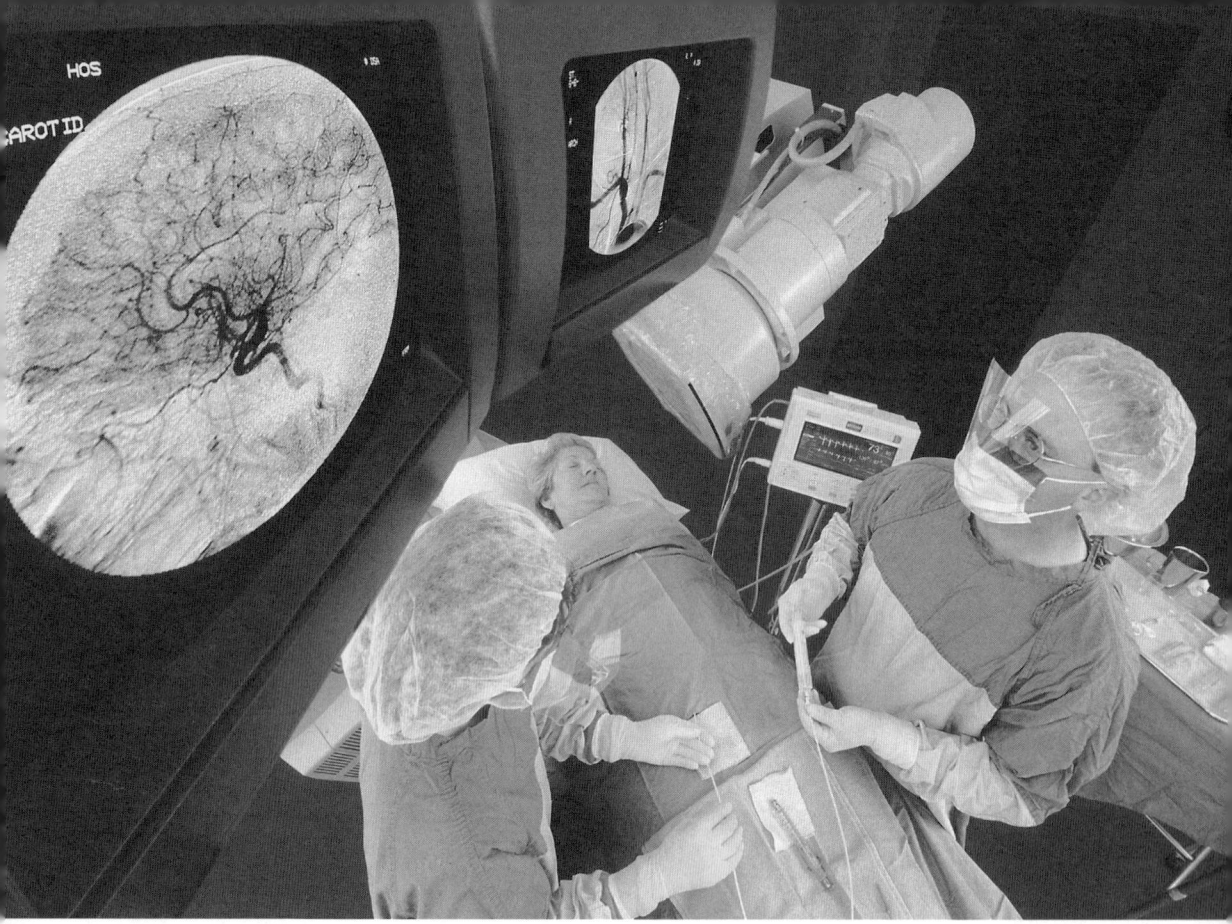

A team of surgeons performs an angiography, an X-ray image of a patient's arteries. X-ray machines provide doctors with precise, three-dimensional images of the human body.

taken of his abdomen to ensure that the bullet had not broken apart and left damaging pieces elsewhere in the president's body. Fortunately, no fragments were found. A short while later Reagan was taken to an operating room for surgery to stop internal bleeding caused by the bullet wound. When Reagan was on the operating table, surgeons had difficulty finding the bullet to remove it. Once more an X-ray was taken, and the position of the bullet was pinpointed within the president's chest. It was finally removed without difficulty, and the bleeding was stopped. President Reagan made a complete recovery and went on to serve two terms in the White House.

Two American presidents, both shot by fanatical gunmen, both with a single bullet lodged in their bodies. Both were immediately attended to by the best physicians available, yet one president dies while the other lives. Although eighty years separated the two shootings, one medical apparatus was common to both: the X-ray machine. Had McKinley's doctors thought to use this new technological device, perhaps the president would have lived. By the time of Reagan's shooting, taking X-rays had become a routine part of medical care, not just for presidents but for the ordinary person as well.

Since the discovery of X-rays at the end of the nineteenth century, this once-mysterious form of radiation has revolutionized the world of medicine, making the diagnosis of illnesses faster and more precise. X-rays have advanced medical knowledge by providing a never-before-available window to the inner workings of the human body. Today, descendants of the first X-ray machines, devices bearing such cryptic names as CT, MRI, and PET, provide strikingly clear views of the body in color and three dimensions. And just as important as their diagnostic function, X-rays are used to fight some of the most dreaded diseases.

With the aid of X-rays, William McKinley might have survived his assassin's bullet, and history would have been forever changed. Without X-rays, Ronald Reagan likely would have succumbed to his would-be assassin's bullet, and history once more would have been different. Today, every person who enters a hospital can benefit from X-rays and other marvels of medical imaging technology.

Chapter 1

Diagnosing Disease

It is often said that the only things certain in life are death and taxes. To this old cliché might be added a third certainty: illness. Disease has been a scourge of the human race from its very beginnings hundreds of thousands of years ago. But only in relatively recent times has humankind developed the skills and the tools to fight, and in many cases conquer, the deadly diseases that are a part of the human condition. Physicians have long struggled with the problem of diagnosing illnesses in their patients, a task made difficult by the healers' understanding, and misunderstanding, of how the human body works.

Diagnosis in History

For centuries, doctors were limited in the methods available to them for diagnosing illnesses in their patients. The simplest method was one that had been used since ancient times: using the five senses to observe changes in the external appearance of a person to determine what was wrong. One medical record from ancient Babylon, for example, contains a description of a patient's symptoms of epilepsy: "At the time of his possession, while he is sitting down, his left eye moves to the side, a lip puckers, saliva flows from his mouth, and his hand, leg, and trunk on the left side jerk like a slaughtered sheep."[1] The use of the word *pos-*

session shows that ancient medicine accepted demons as the cause of many diseases. Ancient physicians had limited means to treat such illnesses, relying mainly on herbal remedies, limited surgical methods, and, as with the epilepsy patient, the driving out of demons by religious "healers."

A new hypothesis for the origin of disease emerged in ancient Greece. This was the theory of "humors" put forth by Hippocrates, a Greek physician who lived from about 460 to 377 B.C. Although Hippocrates is often called "the Father of Medicine," little is actually known about his life and work. But writings attributed to him reveal that he viewed disease as an imbalance of various "humors," or fluids, within the human body. He listed four humors—blood, choler (yellow bile), phlegm, and melancholy (black bile)—that kept the human body alive and determined a person's physical appearance and personality traits. According to this

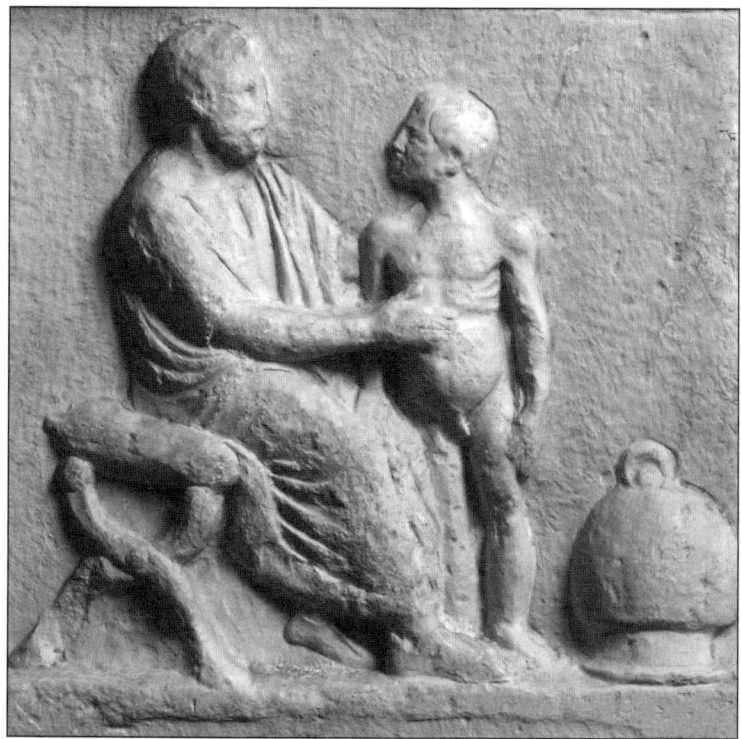

A doctor examines a patient in this ancient Greek relief. External examination was the only diagnostic method available to doctors of the ancient world.

theory, when someone developed too much or too little of one or more of the humors, illness resulted. Hippocrates used close observation of the patient and of the symptoms of illness as his main diagnostic tool. For example, if a patient appeared flushed and feverish, it was thought that too much blood had accumulated in his or her body. The treatment for this condition was to remove the excess blood by bloodletting, a procedure that often killed a patient faster than an illness would have.

Hippocrates acknowledged that diseases were difficult to diagnose and sometimes impossible to cure. However, his view of disease represented a milestone in medical history. It was the antithesis to thousands of years of physicians, priests, and shamans regarding illness as a supernatural visitation upon the victim. Hippocrates viewed disease as a natural occurrence that could be objectively observed and treated. Many historians consider his work as the beginning of scientific medicine, and his theory of humors persisted in medicine into the sixteenth century.

By the seventeenth century, medicine was becoming more scientific, and physicians were learning more about the human body and its inner workings. The body was thought of as a machine, and it was believed to operate in a mechanical way consistent with the laws of physics. No longer was the human body a mysterious entity; instead, it was a mechanism that could be probed, examined, and ultimately understood. Emphasis began to turn from the fluids within the body to a study of the solid organs. Chemistry was also beginning to play a part in the understanding of human physiology, including experiments that revealed the importance of oxygen in sustaining life. The revolutionary theory that blood circulates through the body was put forth by English physician William Harvey, who wrote, "The movement of the blood occurs constantly in a circular manner, and is the result of the beating of the heart."[2] Harvey developed his theory by

Diagnosing Disease

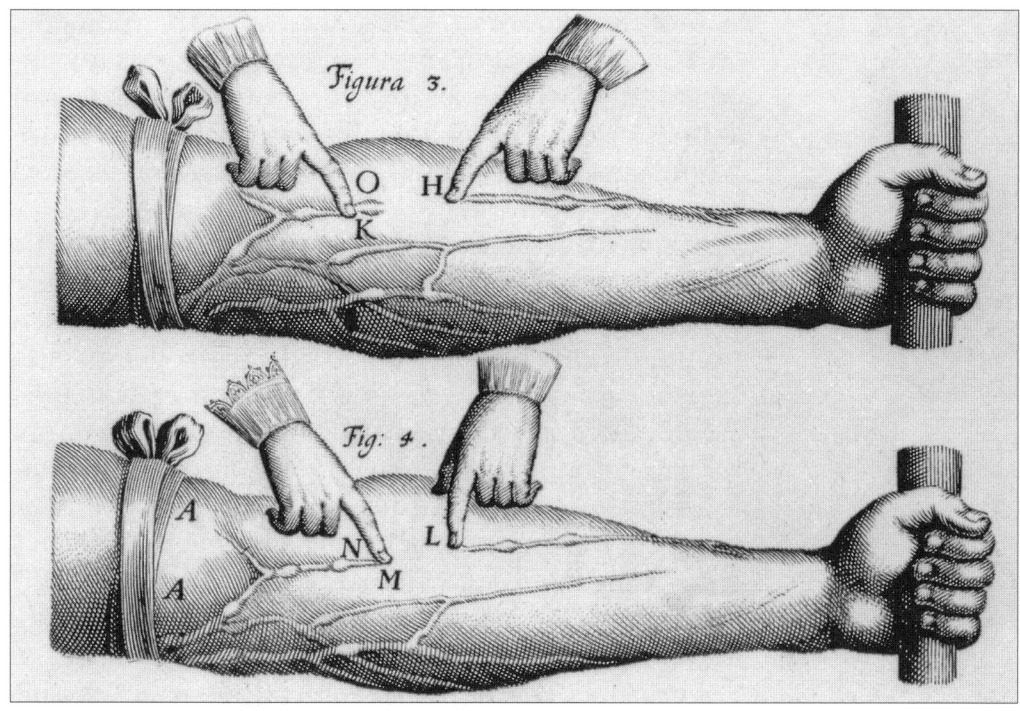

In 1639 William Harvey drew these diagrams showing a forearm tied off with a tourniquet to illustrate the flow of blood through the veins.

carefully observing arteries and veins as they pulsed beneath the skin of his patients.

While scientific progress during the seventeenth century changed the way physicians viewed the human body and its diseases, diagnostic methods remained relatively primitive. But advances in science and technology were poised to enter the field of medicine.

Gauging Temperature

Fever—a rise in body temperature due to the presence of an infection—is one of the most easily discernible symptoms a patient can have. Today's wide variety of thermometers, both modern electronic ones and traditional mercury-filled glass tubes, are familiar instruments in a doctor's bag or home medicine cabinet. But until relatively recently, it was impossible for physicians to determine exactly how high a patient's fever was or whether medications were actually working to reduce the abnormal temperature. The thermometer, an instrument that measures temperature, was invented in the early 1600s by the Italian scientist and astronomer Galileo Galilei. But more than a century would pass before Galileo's instrument would be practical for medical use.

In seventeenth-century Italy, members of scientific circles were pondering the question of how to measure the temperature of the air. Among those who worked on the problem were Galileo and his colleagues in Venice. Today, Galileo is most remembered for the astronomical discoveries he made through the use of his refracting telescope. But among his other scientific achievements was the invention, in 1606, of a thermoscope, the predecessor to the thermometer. Galileo's creation bears little resemblance to modern-day thermometers. It was an egg-shaped glass flask, or bulb, with a tall, thin stem into which water would rise to indicate fluctuations in the temperature of the air. This "air thermometer" was a crude instrument that gave little useful information, and its design made it obviously unsuitable for medical use.

A few years later, a friend of Galileo's named Santorio Santorio modified the thermoscope by adding a numerical scale on which temperatures could be read. Santorio's instrument could be called the first true thermometer since its scale allowed temperatures to be measured. Santorio, who was a physician, then had the idea that the thermometer might be used to measure temperature in his patients. "The patient grasps the bulb," he wrote, "or breathes upon it into a hood, or takes the bulb into his mouth, so that we can tell if the patient is better or worse."[3] Santorio's thermometer allowed him to record changes in a patient's temperature over the course of an illness according to the markings on the instrument's scale. But these markings were arbitrary and held little objective meaning, limiting the thermometer's usefulness.

Diagnosing Disease

About one hundred years after Santorio added his scale to the thermoscope, a Dutch maker of scientific instruments named Daniel Gabriel Fahrenheit devised a more practical scale that standardized temperature readings. This scale, which bears Fahrenheit's name, created a standard for measuring temperature by using two fixed reference points: the temperature of freezing water (30 degrees) and the normal temperature of

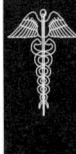

Viewing the Invisible

The microscope, a standard tool of modern-day medical researchers, was first used to view living microorganisms by a seventeenth-century Dutch businessman and amateur scientist named Antoni van Leeuwenhoek. Born in Delft, Holland, in 1632, van Leeuwenhoek became a successful draper, or cloth merchant. In his business, van Leeuwenhoek often used magnifying lenses to determine the quality in the weave of a piece of cloth. But his interest in science led him to explore new ways to use lenses. He became familiar with a simple (single lens) microscope invented by British scientist Robert Hooke, and he soon was constructing his own instruments.

In 1674 van Leeuwenhoek made his greatest discovery. Upon placing some murky lake water under his microscope he was astonished to see tiny creatures swimming in the water. He named these creatures "animalcules," but modern science knows them as bacteria, protozoa, and other microorganisms. He discovered similar creatures in rainwater, well water, and in the human mouth. Van Leeuwenhoek also observed human blood corpuscles and the capillaries that carried them through the body.

Antoni van Leeuwenhoek never made the connection between his little animalcules and disease. But his pioneering studies paved the way for others who would examine blood cells under a microscope to diagnose anemia or observe urine for signs of infection, thus helping to diagnose disease and alleviate suffering.

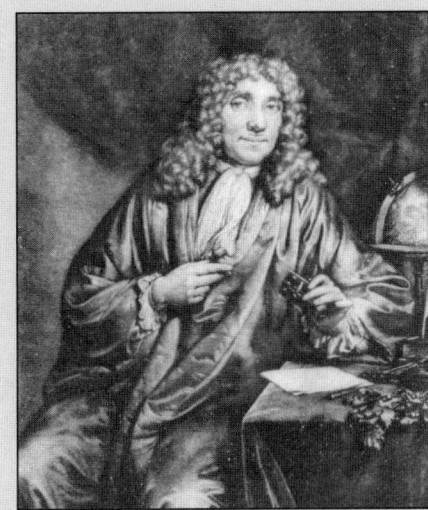

In 1674 Antoni van Leeuwenhoek became the first person to observe microorganisms beneath a microscope.

the human body (90 degrees). These points were later refined to 32 degrees and 98.6 degrees, the marks we are familiar with on modern thermometers. Fahrenheit also was the first to use mercury in a thermometer, a substance he found to have greater sensitivity to temperature changes than water or alcohol had.

Swedish scientist Anders Celsius developed another scale, in which zero degrees is the boiling point of water and one hundred degrees is its freezing point. After his death these points were reversed, resulting in the Celsius scale used today.

Although the addition of mercury and the standardized scales made thermometers more accurate, they were still too cumbersome and slow to register to be useful in medicine. As late as the mid-nineteenth century, thermometers measured over a foot long and sometimes took twenty minutes to display an accurate reading. Around 1866 an English physician named Thomas Allbutt developed the first practical clinical thermometer. Allbutt's thermometer was only about six inches long, and it took a reading in as little as five minutes. It was the true predecessor of our modern mercury thermometers.

Measuring temperature was one way to determine the health of a patient. An even older method made use of the sense of hearing to diagnose illness.

Listening to the Body

Although technology such as the thermometer had begun to enter the field of medicine, physicians were still using antiquated methods of diagnosis. A patient's description of how he or she felt was frequently the major component in diagnosing an illness. This often led to misdiagnosis since many patients may not have been able to accurately describe important symptoms. Observing a patient with the five senses was another diagnostic tool, as it had been since ancient times. Physician and author Stanley Joel Reiser describes how such diagnosis was performed:

The physician focused upon the outward appearance of the patient's body, mainly the facial expression, posture, tongue, skin color, and manner of breathing. He also examined the appearance of the blood, urine, and stools. A third method of examination used to judge the presence of disease—and the method least used—was the physical examination of the body. At this period the physician's only tool was his sense of touch. He used it most often to feel the pulse and estimate its quality, without determining its exact rate. He used a sense of touch somewhat less frequently to judge the body's temperature, and occasionally to detect tenderness or abnormal masses by briskly probing the tissues beneath the skin.[4]

Greek physician Hippocrates knew the value of listening to the sounds in a patient's chest to detect disease, a process known as auscultation. "You shall know by this," he wrote, "that the chest contains water or pus, if in applying the ear during a certain time on the side, you perceive a noise like that of boiling vinegar."[5] In the eighteenth century a Viennese doctor named Leopold Auenbrugger von Auenbrugg developed a method called percussion as a means of diagnosis. Using percussion entailed a physician lightly tapping a patient's chest and listening to the resulting tone. The pitch of the sound indicated the presence or absence of fluid in the lungs, thus aiding in the diagnosis of chest and lung diseases. Auenbrugger is often credited as being the founder of physical diagnosis as a science. The problem with using human senses such as hearing to aid in diagnosis, however, is that they are not sensitive enough to determine exactly what is going on inside the human body. In the nineteenth century a young French doctor with a long name invented a device that helped revolutionize medical diagnosis.

René-Théophile-Hyacinthe Laënnec was a physician at the Necker Hospital in Paris in the early nineteenth century. He knew of Hippocrates' method of listening to a patient's chest, and he had even tried it himself, with disappointing results. Not only was it difficult to discern any sounds of disease, but modesty made it embarrassing for a physician to place his ear directly on a patient, especially if the patient was female.

One day in 1816, Laënnec faced a problem while examining a rather obese woman who had a heart ailment. The woman's size, as well as her sex, prohibited Laënnec from placing his ear on her chest to listen to her heart. While pondering this dilemma, Laënnec remembered recently watching some children at play. He recalled how one child would tap a nail at one end of a long wooden board while a child at the opposite end listened, delighted at how the tiny sound of the nail was easily heard. Of course, it was simple physics: Sound is amplified when it travels through physical objects. Laënnec rolled several sheets of paper into a cylinder and placed one end on the patient's chest. When he put his ear to the other end, the sounds of the woman's heart came through clearly. "From this moment," he wrote, "I imagined that the circumstance might furnish means for enabling us to ascertain the character, not only of the action of the heart, but of every species of sound produced by the motion of all the thoracic viscera [internal organs]."[6]

Laënnec called his invention a stethoscope, from the Greek words *stethos* ("chest"), and *scope* ("to view"). It revolutionized the art of diagnosing chest and heart diseases. For the next three years he refined his design,

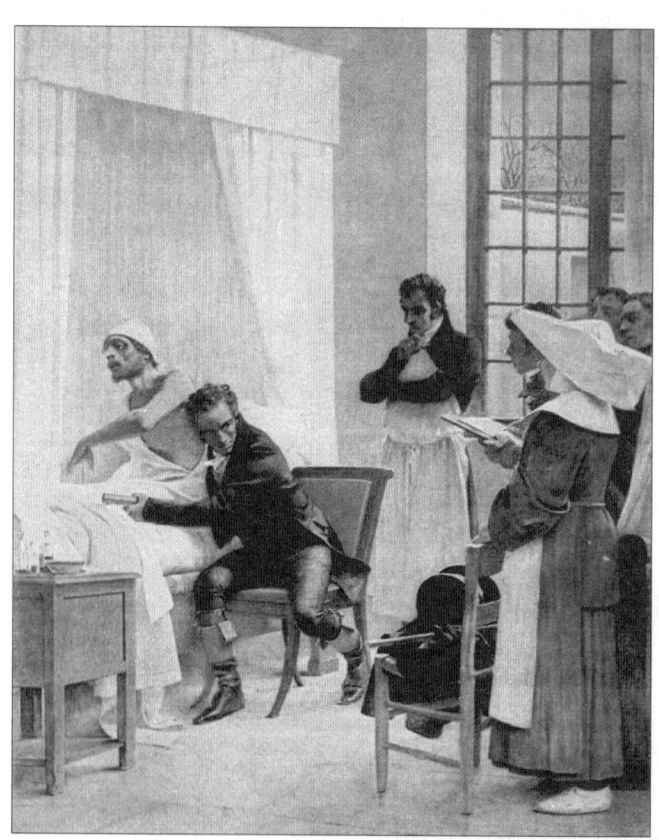

René Laënnec places his ear at a patient's chest to listen to his heart. In 1816 Laënnec invented the stethoscope, a device that revolutionized the art of diagnosing chest and heart disease.

finally settling on a hollow wooden cylinder about nine inches long. In 1819 Laënnec wrote a treatise for physicians entitled *On Mediate Auscultation*, which explained how to diagnose various illnesses using his stethoscope. Although Laënnec died early, at age forty-five in 1826, his invention spread throughout the medical community. By the mid-1800s Laënnec's hollow wooden cylinder had evolved into a device with two flexible rubber tubes that allowed listening with both ears—the binaural stethoscope we are familiar with today.

Hearing was not the only sense physicians used to detect illnesses in their patients. The sense of sight would prove to be even more valuable in the realm of medical diagnostics.

Looking Within

In observing a patient's physical appearance during a medical examination, doctors in the seventeenth and eighteenth centuries were utilizing a method of diagnosis as old as Hippocrates himself. As might be expected with any medical procedure having ancient roots, observation had its limitations. Physicians could only see the external condition of a patient, and thus had to rely on obvious physical symptoms to assist them in making a diagnosis. Stanley Joel Reiser notes that the "physician focused upon the outward appearance of the patient's body, mainly the facial expression, posture, tongue, skin color, and manner of breathing."[7] The useful results of such observation were rather limited and had to be augmented by the patient's own description of his or her symptoms for even a cursory diagnosis to be made. The ability to see inside the body to observe the workings, and malfunctions, of the various organs would have greatly increased the accuracy of the diagnostic process. But at the time, the only method available for observing the interior of the living human body was through surgery, which was both risky and painful for the patient. Autopsies, of course, allowed doctors to study the insides of a deceased patient, but this obviously came too late to help the poor departed soul.

All this changed in the nineteenth century, however, as physicians sought ways to see into the living bodies of their patients. It is fitting that these advances first took place in ophthalmology, the study of diseases of the eye.

Inventing the Ophthalmoscope

Hermann von Helmholtz was a nineteenth-century German physicist and mathematician. His many scientific interests included heat, acoustics, electricity and magnetism, and the conservation of energy. Trained as a surgeon, Helmholtz later went into research and became the first person to measure the speed of nerve impulses. In 1850 his studies of optics led him to conduct experiments on how light enters, and is reflected by, the human eye. For these experiments he needed an instrument that would allow him to observe the interior of the eye while illuminating it with a candle or small lamp. He realized that in order to do this, he would have to place his eye at the same point from which the light was shining. For a week Helmholtz tinkered with various methods to accomplish this task. The instrument he finally developed, which he called the ophthalmoscope, was a small handheld device that featured a piece of glass mounted at a forty-five-degree angle and, behind it, a lens. An external light was bounced off the glass and into the patient's eye. The physician, looking through the lens of the instrument, could observe the interior of the eye from the reflected light rays passing back through the glass.

The ophthalmoscope revolutionized the diagnosis of eye diseases. Now physicians could see for themselves the inner structure of the eye, described in a medical journal of Helmholtz's day as a "spectacle of the red vessels on the transparent white ground"[8] of the retina. There were some initial fears that the new instrument actually caused certain eye disorders, including blindness, rather than revealed them. But

Diagnosing Disease

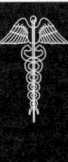

A Window into the Body

In 1822 a freak hunting accident provided a military doctor with a unique opportunity to view the inner workings of a living human body. On June 6 of that year, a twenty-eight-year-old fur trapper named Alexis St. Martin suffered an accidental musket wound in his abdomen in northern Michigan. William Beaumont, a U.S. Army physician stationed on an island in Lake Michigan, treated the injury and saved St. Martin's life. But the wound failed to heal completely, leaving a permanent hole in St. Martin's abdomen.

Beaumont realized that he could learn about the human digestive system by observing St. Martin's stomach through the "window" in his abdomen. In 1825 Beaumont began a series of historic experiments. He observed the actions of gastric juices on different types of foods and studied the effects of weather, stress, and stomach temperature on the digestive process. In 1833 Beaumont published his findings in a book entitled *Experiments and Observations on the Gastric Juice and the Physiology of Digestion.*

Alexis St. Martin lived for fifty-eight years after his accidental wounding. He died in Canada on June 24, 1880. A plaque near his grave reminds visitors that "through his affliction he served all humanity."

Doctor William Beaumont treats a musket wound in the abdomen of a young fur trapper.

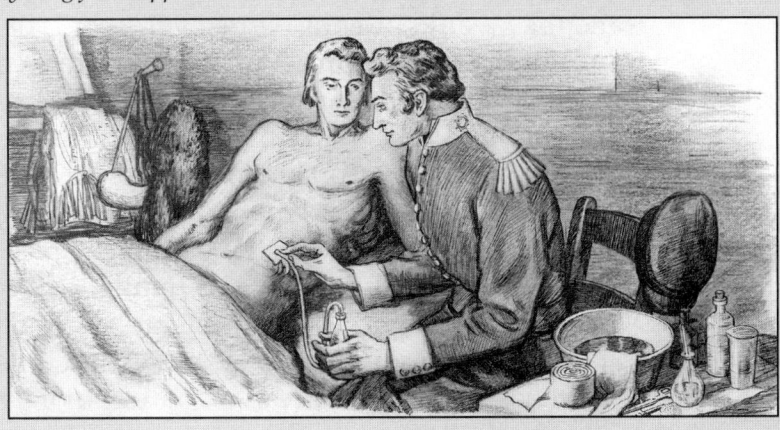

these fears proved unfounded, and physicians soon embraced the use of Helmholtz's invention. By 1855 the ophthalmoscope had crossed the Atlantic and was being used by doctors in the United States.

For the first time it was possible to see inside a living body, even though it was just a small part of it. The invention of the ophthalmoscope spurred medical researchers to devise optical means to observe the inside of other body cavities. Instruments called endoscopes were invented to examine the sinuses, larynx, esophagus, stomach, and colon. By the 1870s these instruments were equipped with electric lights in order to illuminate the internal cavities and make the tissues and their disorders more easily discernible to physicians.

Another nineteenth-century invention seemed, at first, to hold promise as a tool in diagnostics: photography.

Medical Imaging

Medical illustration, the art of depicting human anatomy, can, in a sense, trace its roots back to ancient times, when cave dwellers drew human figures on cave walls. By the 1850s photography, which had been invented earlier in the nineteenth century, was thought to have some promise as a tool in medicine. For example, photographs could illustrate the appearance of illnesses more objectively than a doctor could describe them, and they would provide permanent records of diseases and surgical procedures. But several factors combined to slow the acceptance of photography in medicine. The primitive cameras of the day were large and cumbersome, and they required long exposure times to take a picture. Photographs had to be made on fragile glass plates that required messy, dangerous chemicals to prepare them for exposure. In addition, it took considerable skill and experience to master the technology and art of photography. Because of these difficulties, interest in using photography as a medical tool waned.

In the late nineteenth century photography had made great advances in both the quality of photographs and the ease with which they could be taken. Cameras were smaller and easier to use, exposure times were shorter, and celluloid film had replaced glass plates and chemicals for recording images. Interest in capturing the human anatomy on film was once again on the rise. Despite the technical advances in photography, however, pictures could still show only the exterior of the human body; there was no way for the camera to peer inside a patient to aid in diagnosing an illness. But research was already under way in Europe that would soon lead to the breakthrough of capturing images of the inside of the body. These experiments were being carried out by physicists attempting to discover the nature of invisible particles emitted by powerful electric currents.

Chapter 2
Wilhelm Röntgen's "New Rays"

Bertha Röntgen was worried. For months her husband, Wilhelm, had been acting in a very peculiar manner. He was spending almost all of his waking hours in his laboratory at the University of Würzburg in Germany. Röntgen's workrooms were on the first floor of the university's Physical Science Institute; he and Bertha lived in a small apartment on the institute's second floor. Röntgen was usually late for supper, and when he finally came home for meals, he sat sullenly at the table, eating little of the food Bertha had prepared. Then it was back to the laboratory for more work, often late into the night. Bertha had no idea what was wrong with her husband, for her inquiries about his work went unanswered.

In time, Bertha would come to understand her husband's strange behavior. But for now, Wilhelm Conrad Röntgen worked alone on a discovery that would change the world of medical diagnosis.

A Persistent Student

Röntgen (also spelled Roentgen) was born in Lennep, Prussia (now Remscheid, Germany), on March 27, 1845, the only child of Friedrich and Charlotte Röntgen, the owners of a textile mill. Wilhelm enjoyed a happy and carefree youth, receiving his early education at private schools in Holland, where his family moved when he was three years old. Young Wilhelm demonstrated a love of the outdoors and an aptitude for making mechanical devices. A promising future seemed assured for the young man, until he was expelled from his gymnasium, the European term for high school, when he was seventeen. One day in 1862 a classmate at the gymnasium had drawn a caricature of a teacher on the blackboard. As Wilhelm was admiring this humorous artwork, the teacher walked in. When asked who had made the drawing, Wilhelm remained silent, refusing to betray his classmate. The punishment for his recalcitrance was severe: Wilhelm was expelled from the gymnasium.

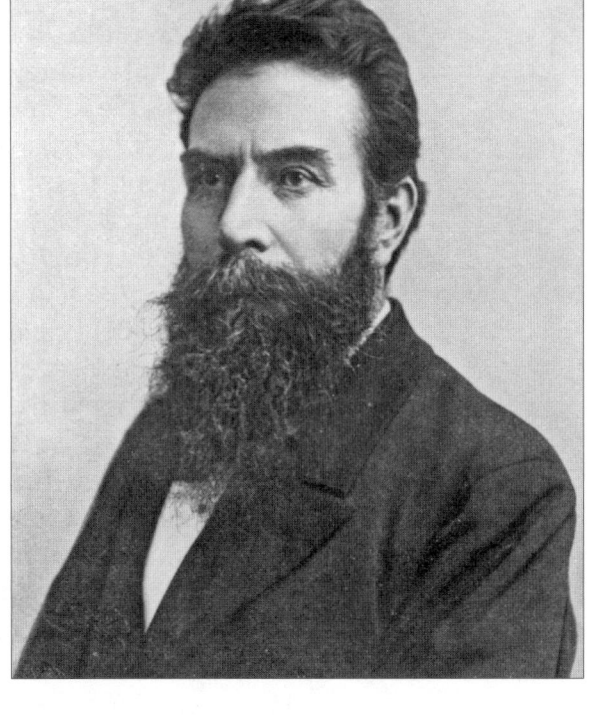

Wilhelm Röntgen's 1895 discovery of X-rays was one of the most important advancements in the history of medicine.

Graduation from gymnasium was required for students planning further education at a university in Holland or Germany, and it now looked as if Wilhelm would never achieve that goal. But he found a way to further his education by studying with private tutors and taking university courses for no credit. "In order not to lose touch with science," Röntgen wrote, "I registered myself as an auditor at Utrecht University. There I attended lectures on physics, chemistry, and zoology."[9] In 1865 he entered the Polytechnic in Zurich, Switzerland, a technical school that did not require a *matura*, or diploma, from a gymnasium. At the Polytechnic, Röntgen studied mechanical engineering and received his degree in that field in 1868. But he was uncertain what direction his life should take. Persuaded by a professor to continue his education, he began studies in physics. "My old love for physics was born anew," he wrote. Although he could not enroll as a regular university student without a *matura*, he knew that "it was possible for me, according to the rules, to obtain my degree if I could produce a sufficiently good thesis on a scientific subject."[10] Röntgen polished up and then submitted a research paper on gases that he had written at the Polytechnic. Based on this work, the young man who had been denied a gymnasium diploma received his PhD in physics in 1869.

Over the next several years, Wilhelm Röntgen held academic posts at the Universities of Würzburg and Strasbourg, and in 1879 he began a tenure at the University of Giessen. In 1872 Röntgen had married Anna Bertha Ludwig, the attractive daughter of a Zurich innkeeper. The couple lived a happy life, even though Bertha suffered from lingering, probably psychosomatic illnesses. On their yearly hiking vacations to Switzerland, Röntgen could usually be found taking photographs of the scenery. Although the cameras of the day were heavy and cumbersome, he was meticulous about visually documenting his travels. Photographic plates of the kind Röntgen used on vacation would later play a role in the development of X-rays as a diagnostic tool.

After spending nine years teaching physics at the University of Giessen, Röntgen returned to the University of Würzburg, this time as a professor of theoretical physics. Although a rather dry and uninspiring lecturer, Röntgen nonetheless captivated his students with his experiments and demonstrations. In 1894, after six years as a professor at Würzburg, he became the rector, or head, of the university. But in his heart he was still an experimental physicist, proclaiming to an assembly gathered at the university that "the experiment is still the most powerful and the most reliable lever enabling us to extract secrets from nature."[11] Röntgen would indeed extract the X-ray from nature, but his discovery would build upon the work of other physicists.

William Crookes's Tube

While Wilhelm Röntgen was teaching at the University of Würzburg, a scientist in England was performing experiments using a special kind of glass tube that he had developed. William Crookes devoted his life to performing research in chemistry and physics. He discovered a new element, which he named thallium, and invented the radiometer, an instrument for measuring radiant energy. In the late nineteenth century Crookes was conducting experiments with powerful electric currents. As other physicists had already discovered, passing a high-voltage electric charge through a glass tube from which most of the air had been evacuated (vacuum tube) caused the walls of the tube to glow. No one understood what caused this glow, and Crookes was among the many scientists trying to find out.

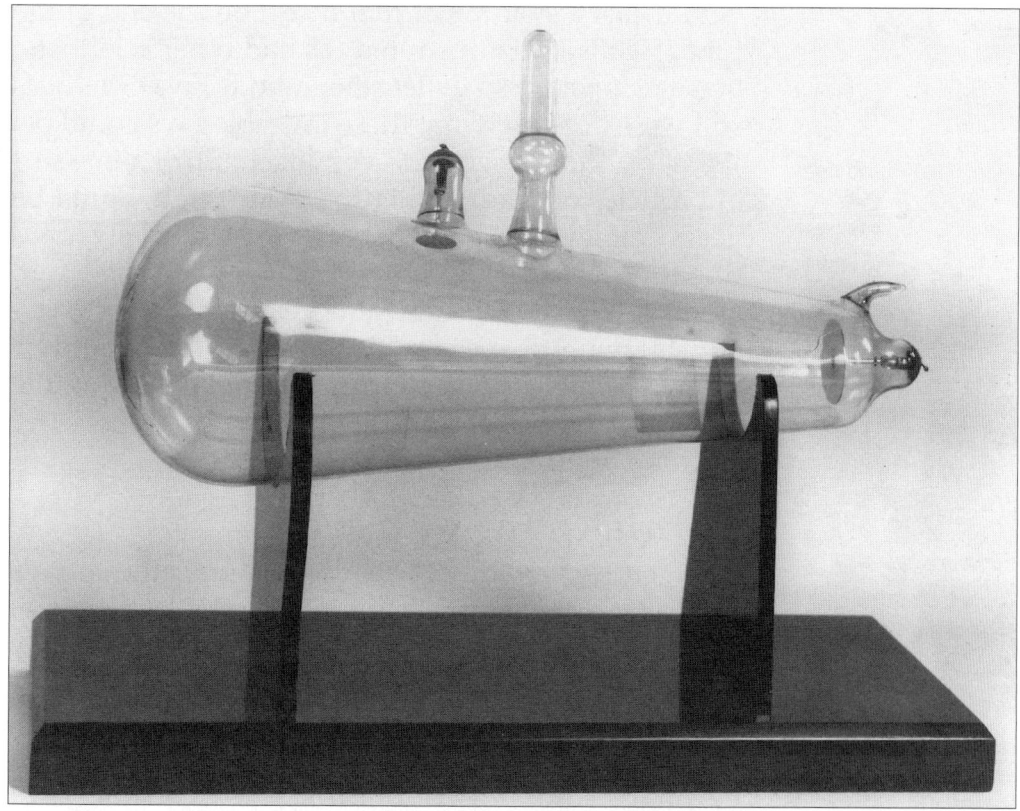

This cylindrical glass tube known as a Crookes tube is similar to those Röntgen used in his X-ray experiments.

Most vacuum tubes of the time were either cylindrical or globe shaped. For Crookes's experiments, he created a tube that was more efficient than any previous design. Named the Crookes tube after its inventor, the device looked like a large pear-shaped light bulb. At one end of the tube was a metal plate known as a cathode; another metal plate, the anode, entered the tube from the side. When a high-voltage generator was attached to the plates, an invisible current passed through the vacuum between the metal plates. Since this current originated at the cathode and flowed in a straight line similar to rays of visible light, it became known as cathode rays.

Sometimes, however, some of the cathode rays would miss the anode and strike the walls of the tube, causing them to fluoresce, or glow. When Crookes placed a thin piece of metal inside the tube, the rays would cast a shadow of that object on the end of the tube. He also demonstrated (as had other scientists) that a magnet could deflect the cathode rays. Scientists still were not sure what these invisible rays could be. Were they composed of waves, like light, or some sort of particles or "radiant matter"? (In fact, it would be years before these cathode rays were accurately identified as electrons, the negatively charged particles in atoms.) Crookes tubes became very popular with scientists trying to answer this question. They could be found in laboratories all over Europe, including the laboratory of Wilhelm Röntgen at the Physical Science Institute of the University of Würzburg.

Experimenting with Rays

Röntgen was aware of the research on cathode rays being conducted by other European scientists. The subject was especially intriguing to physicists in Germany and England, who debated the composition of the mysterious cathode rays. As many researchers did when embarking on a new field of investigation, Röntgen began his studies by duplicating the experiments of others. By using his acute powers of observation, he felt that he might uncover some new phenomenon that earlier scientists had overlooked. "Roentgen was a genius of interpretation of phenomena," a colleague wrote, "had a keen sense of observation, and an inexhaustible thoroughness of critical judgment, combined with brilliant experimental skill."[12]

In June 1895 Röntgen began his experiments in his laboratory on the first floor of the Physical Science Institute. In the small lab were several wooden shelves and tables filled with the instruments necessary for investigating cathode rays: a device called a Ruhmkorff coil that produced high-voltage electrical current, numerous glass tubes in various sizes and shapes, and a vacuum pump to evacuate the air from the tubes. As he was a skilled mechanic, Röntgen had constructed

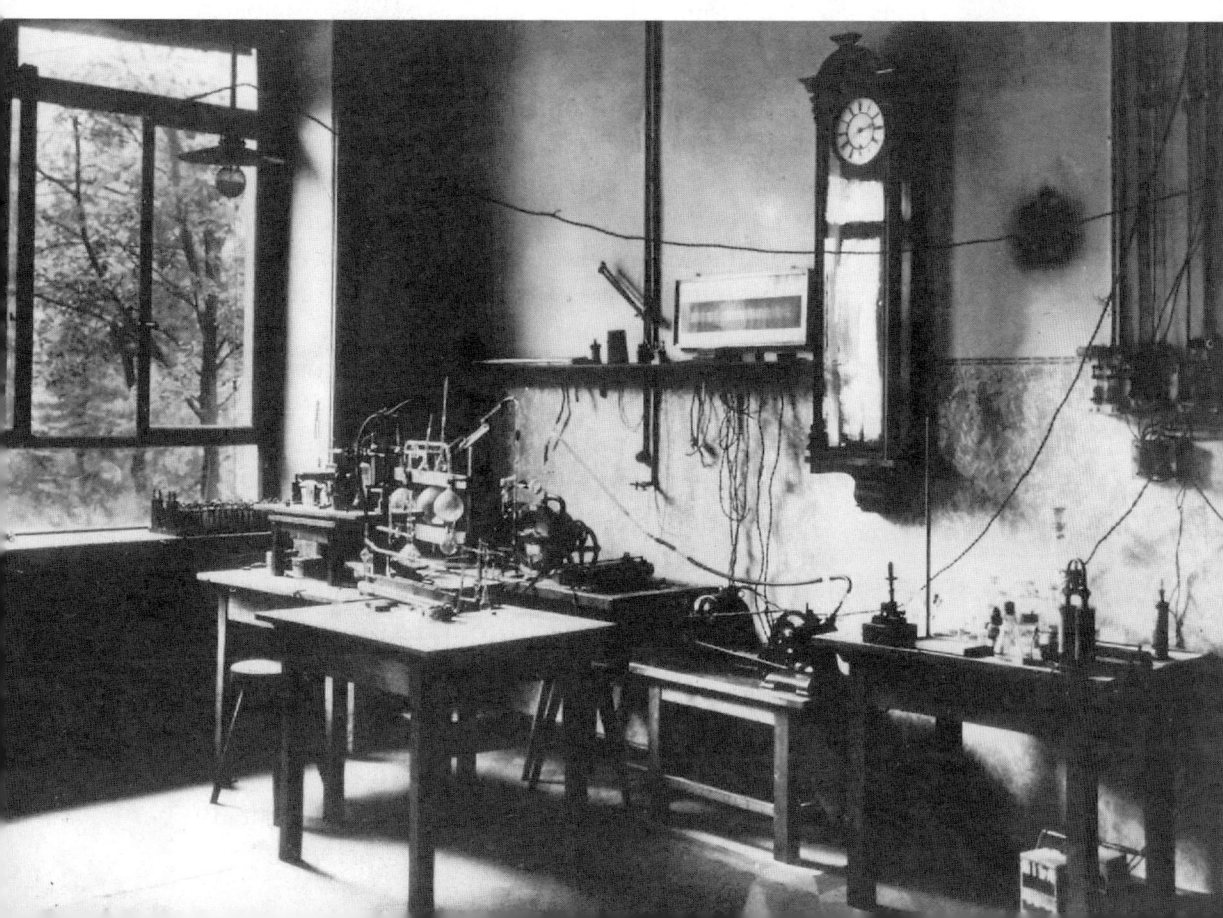

Röntgen spent many long days inside this laboratory at the University of Würzburg, Germany, where he researched the properties of cathode rays.

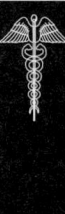

A Scientific Obsession

Wilhelm Conrad Röntgen's discovery of X-rays in November 1895 quickly turned from a scientific inquiry into an obsession. Everything—including friends, other research projects, meals, and even his own wife—suddenly became secondary to his study of the new rays. Before he could announce his discovery to the world, Röntgen had to convince himself that X-rays were real. W. Robert Nitske's book The Life of Wilhelm Conrad Röntgen, Discoverer of the X Ray, *includes Röntgen's own account of his preoccupation with X-rays.*

When at first I made the startling discovery of the penetrating rays, it was such an extraordinary astonishing phenomenon that I had to convince myself repeatedly by doing the same experiment over and over and over again to make absolutely certain that the rays actually existed. I was not aware of anything else but the strange phenomenon in the laboratory. Was it a fact or an illusion? I was torn between doubt and hope, and did not want to have any other thoughts interfere with my experiments. I tried to exclude everything not pertinent to the laboratory work from my thinking. Any interference could have caused me to fail in the creation of identical conditions to substantiate the discovery. I made the observations many, many times before I was able to accept the phenomenon myself. During those trying days I was in a state of shock.

many of the instruments himself. Two large windows admitted ample daylight into the room, and a stove provided heat during the cold winter months. Compared to the great laboratories at other European universities, it was a modest setting for a major scientific discovery. "The lesson of the laboratory was eloquent," wrote reporter H.J.W. Dam, who visited Röntgen's lab shortly after his discovery. "It mutely said that in the great march of science it is the genius of man, not the perfection of appliances that breaks new ground in the great territory of the unknown."[13]

Before long, Röntgen became so obsessed with cathode rays that he abandoned his other studies to devote all his time to experimenting with them. For months he passed electric currents through tubes of various sizes and shapes, observing the fluorescence that glowed on the walls of the tubes. Often he found that the tubes he had purchased were insufficiently evacuated, so he devised a way to precisely control the amount of air removed from a tube. As Röntgen methodically performed his experiments, he confirmed the observations of other scientists who had previously studied cathode rays. One physicist whose work Röntgen repeated was Philipp Lenard. Lenard's experiments showed that cathode rays could escape a vacuum tube through an aluminum-covered window in the side of the tube. Since cathode rays are invisible, Lenard coated a small cardboard screen with a chemical called barium platinocyanide. When cathode rays struck the screen, they caused the chemical to glow, proving that the rays had indeed traveled through the window. The screen had to be placed very close to the window, however, because cathode rays could go only a few centimeters through air.

Röntgen's experiments confirmed what Lenard and other scientists already knew, but they did not add any new knowledge to the field. It was not until a cold Friday in November that Röntgen made his fortuitous discovery.

Röntgen's Discovery

Alone in his laboratory on the afternoon of November 8, 1895, Röntgen began an experiment using a Crookes tube. He had duplicated Lenard's results, but now he wanted to find out if cathode rays could escape a vacuum tube that did not have an aluminum window. In order to see the faint glow of a barium platinocyanide screen that would confirm or refute his results, the laboratory needed to be pitch black. Roentgen drew the curtains over the room's windows. Then he carefully covered the Crookes tube with pieces of black cardboard so that the fluorescence from inside the tube would not escape and spoil the darkness of the room. When he was satisfied that the tube was completely shielded, he turned off the laboratory's lights and switched on the Ruhmkorff coil, sending high-voltage current through the Crookes tube. The familiar odor of ozone, produced by the electrical current, filled the laboratory.

As he was examining the tube to make sure no light was leaking from beneath the cardboard cover, something caught his attention. Out of the corner of his eye he thought he saw the glimmer of illumination in the darkened room. He turned to look at the strange light and there, across the laboratory, he indeed saw a flickering glow. The light was a greenish yellow color, but because Röntgen was partially colorblind, he noticed only the brightness. This was peculiar, Röntgen thought. With the lights off and the curtains drawn, there was no source of illumination in the laboratory that could be creating the strange luminescence. By the light of a match, Röntgen discovered that the glow came from a barium platinocyanide screen he had been using in his experiments. But why was the screen glowing? Something was obviously amiss, and Röntgen was determined to find out what it was.

He decided to check his apparatus again. When he turned off the Ruhmkorff coil, to his astonishment, the glow disappeared. Now thoroughly puzzled, Röntgen restarted the coil and the glow returned. Several times he turned the electricity off and on, and each time that the Crookes tube was energized, the strange light returned. It appeared that the rays from the Crookes tube were somehow striking the cardboard screen, causing it to fluoresce. Röntgen knew from duplicating Lenard's experiments that cathode rays could only travel a few centimeters outside a vacuum tube. But the screen that was now glowing sat on a table several feet from the energized tube, too far for the cathode rays to be the cause of the illumination. The Crookes tube was apparently producing some other type of rays along with the familiar cathode rays. Since he knew nothing about these new rays, he called them X-rays—
X being the scientific notation for something unknown.

For the next several days Röntgen performed numerous experiments to try to determine the nature of this strange new phenomenon. One of the interesting things he discovered about X-rays was their ability to penetrate solid objects. When he placed a one-thousand-page book between the Crookes tube and the barium platinocyanide screen, the X-rays passed through the book with just a slight dimming of the fluorescent screen. A double deck of playing cards produced the same results. Röntgen experimented with a variety of materials: paper, wood, glass, rubber, and many different kinds of metal. The X-rays easily passed through almost every object that Röntgen placed in front of the tube. Several metals, however, were able to stop the rays, in varying degrees. A single piece of tinfoil was transparent to the rays, but several sheets folded together produced a shadow on the screen, evidence that the X-rays were being partially blocked. Thin sheets of aluminum, gold, copper, and platinum allowed some X-rays to pass through, while lead stopped the rays completely. While performing his experiments, Röntgen made

How X-rays Work

The atom, once thought to be the smallest building block of matter, is actually made up of even smaller particles known as protons, neutrons, and electrons. Protons and neutrons reside in the center, or nucleus, of the atom, while electrons whirl in orbits, like tiny satellites, around the nucleus. These orbiting electrons are what make technology such as radio, television, and X-rays possible.

Every vacuum tube contains a negative electrode, called the cathode, and a positive electrode, called the anode. When electricity is applied to the tube, electrons are released from their orbits around the atoms of the cathode. These free electrons can perform various tasks as they speed through the vacuum of the tube. To create an X-ray picture, electrons leave the cathode and strike the anode (sometimes called the "anticathode"), producing high-energy electromagnetic radiation called X-rays. These rays leave the tube through a window built into the tube's protective lead shield. An object, such as a human body, placed between the window and a piece of photographic film, will block the X-rays in varying degrees. When the film is developed, dense areas will show up as light spots, and other, less dense areas will remain dark. By studying these films doctors can examine breaks in bones, discover foreign objects in the body, and diagnose tumors that may indicate a life-threatening disease.

Wilhelm Conrad Röntgen knew nothing of electrons when he made his famous discovery in 1895. But the X-rays created by those electrons have become a vital diagnostic instrument for physicians, dentists, and other healthcare professionals.

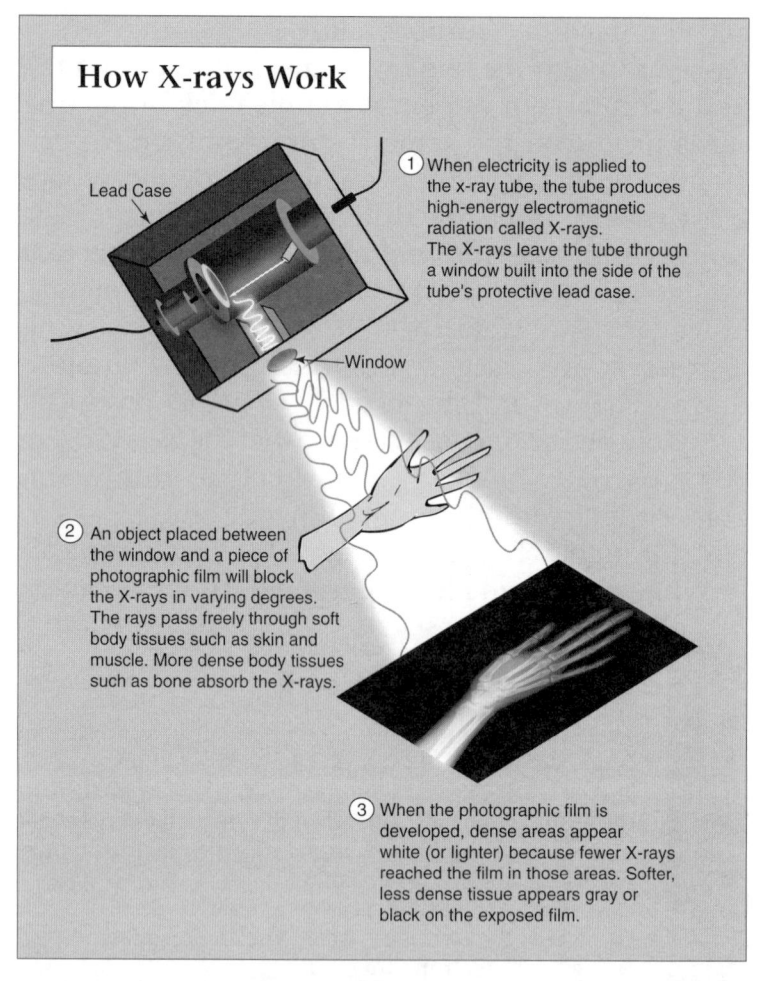

How X-rays Work

① When electricity is applied to the x-ray tube, the tube produces high-energy electromagnetic radiation called X-rays. The X-rays leave the tube through a window built into the side of the tube's protective lead case.

② An object placed between the window and a piece of photographic film will block the X-rays in varying degrees. The rays pass freely through soft body tissues such as skin and muscle. More dense body tissues such as bone absorb the X-rays.

③ When the photographic film is developed, dense areas appear white (or lighter) because fewer X-rays reached the film in those areas. Softer, less dense tissue appears gray or black on the exposed film.

a discovery that was both amazing and disturbing. As he held various items between the tube and the screen, he was startled to see the dark shadows of the bones in his hand projected on the screen. The X-rays were partially blocked by the bones beneath living human flesh, resulting in a ghostly image of the inside of Röntgen's hand.

Photographing the Invisible

To obtain a permanent record of his experiments, Röntgen began substituting unexposed photographic plates for the barium platinocyanide screen. When developed, these X-rays became photographic negatives, showing white spaces where the rays had been stopped and gray or black areas where the rays went through. Printing the negatives reversed the light and dark spaces of the images. These X-ray photographs proved to Röntgen once and for all that he was not observing just an optical illusion. "I found by accident," he later commented, "that the rays penetrated black paper. I then used wood, paper, books, but I still believed I was the victim of deception. Finally, I used photography and the experiment was successfully culminated."[14]

Tired of always having to black out his entire laboratory for his experiments, Röntgen decided to simplify the process. So he built a "darkroom," a lightproof

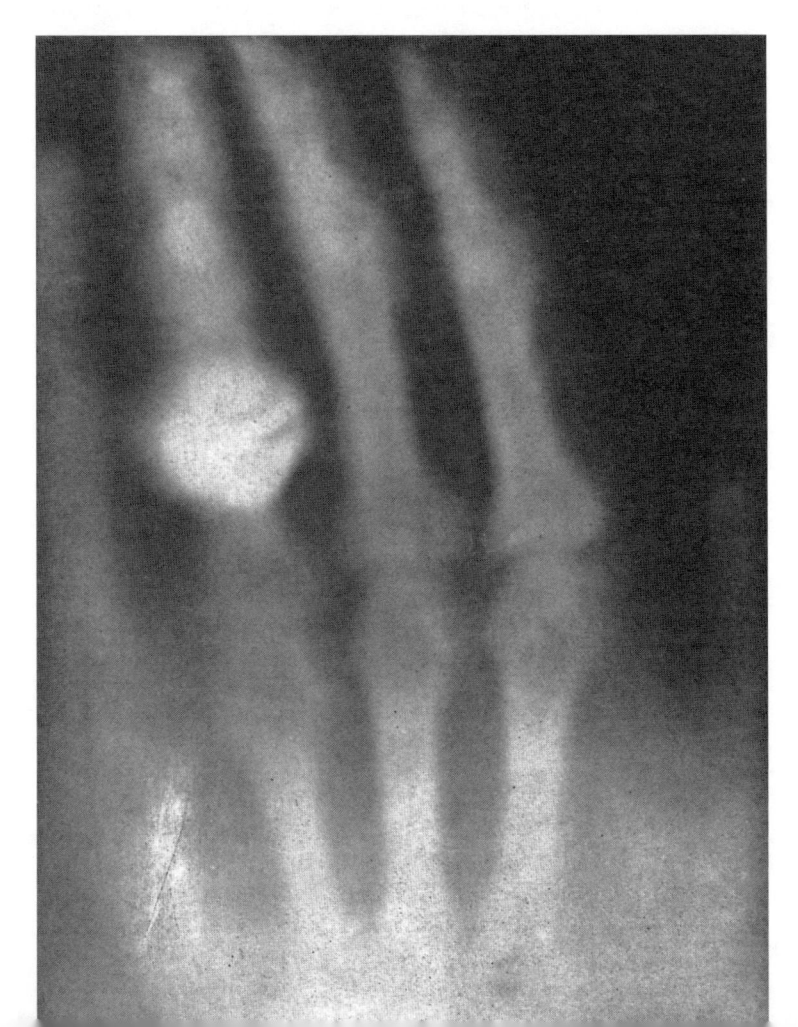

In December 1895 Röntgen made this X-ray image of his wife's hand, revealing her bones and a ring on her finger.

(and X-ray–proof) box large enough for him to step inside. The Crookes tube remained outside, with the X-rays entering the box through a circular opening covered with aluminum. To perform an experiment, Röntgen had only to enter the box with his materials and close the door behind him. The many images Röntgen made during his experimenting included X-ray photographs of metal weights inside a wooden box, a compass whose dial markings had been painted with lead paint, and even his shotgun. When he tried to take X-ray photographs through his laboratory door, he was puzzled by the appearance of light strips on the photographs. Röntgen finally realized that the strips were caused by lead paint on the door, which blocked the X-rays.

Röntgen worked alone in strict secrecy, telling his two laboratory assistants nothing of his investigations. Even his wife, Bertha, remained mystified as to why her husband suddenly had become sullen and uncommunicative. He did make a vague remark to his close friend, Theodor Boveri, who had become concerned about Röntgen's sudden change in personality. "I have discovered something interesting," Röntgen told him, "but I don't know whether or not my observations are correct."[15] Finally, after six weeks of intensive experimentation, Röntgen was ready to explain to Bertha what had been consuming all his time and attention.

On December 22, 1895, Röntgen led his wife down to his laboratory. He showed Bertha the Crookes tube and explained its operation. Then he asked her to place her hand on an unexposed photographic plate that he had placed on a table under the tube. After energizing the tube for fifteen minutes, Röntgen developed the film and showed Bertha the result. There, on the film, was the outline of Bertha's bones, with her rings showing up as a dark spot on her third finger. Bertha's reaction was not one of delight, as Röntgen had hoped, but of alarm and fear. Seeing her bones was, to Bertha, a premonition of her own approaching death. It was nothing of the sort, as she would live to the age of eighty, but her reaction was not uncommon among people who would later view X-ray photographs of their bones. The photograph of Bertha's hand, however, would become a familiar sight when Röntgen finally decided to tell the world of his discovery.

"A New Kind of Rays"

Once a scientist makes a significant discovery, the next step is usually to publish his findings in a scientific journal in order to be credited with that discovery. Throughout his weeks of concentrated experimenting, Röntgen had kept his work on X-rays to himself. Now that he had told Bertha, he felt the time was right to share his breakthrough with the scientific world. But time was also his adversary, for he needed to publish quickly lest other scientists who were experimenting with cathode rays make the same discovery he had. Indeed, for all he knew, someone may have already duplicated his findings and was preparing to publish.

He assembled his notes and immediately began to set down the details of his experiments. Writing quickly and economically by hand, Röntgen included "not a single word not imposed by absolute necessity."[16] On December 28, 1895, Röntgen's initial report was finished. Titled "A New Kind of Rays" (also referred to as the Preliminary, or First, Communication), the paper detailed Röntgen's experiments and how the X-rays acted on the various materials he had placed in front of the Crookes tube. Röntgen hand delivered the paper to the president of the Physico-Medical Society in Würzburg, to be published in the society's journal. Although such papers are usually read aloud at scientific society meetings, there had been no meeting that December. Nonetheless, the president recognized the importance of Röntgen's discovery, and the society immediately published the paper. Röntgen was officially on record as the discoverer of X-rays.

> ## Who Really Discovered X-rays?
>
> Wilhelm Conrad Röntgen is universally recognized as the discoverer of X-rays. But was he really the first to create this important phenomenon? The record of history shows that he was not.
>
> A few years before Röntgen's discovery, physicist Philipp Lenard noticed that a barium platinocyanide–coated paper glowed when he energized a vacuum tube during an experiment. Although it was this same phenomenon that sparked Röntgen's investigations into X-rays, Lenard did not think to pursue it. When Röntgen announced his discovery, Lenard became jealous, feeling that he had actually observed X-rays first. His resentment was so strong that Lenard refused to use the term *X-rays*, preferring to call the phenomenon wave radiation instead. X-rays were also known as Röntgen rays, which must have particularly infuriated Lenard. He halfheartedly tried to explain his claim of priority, quoted here from W. Robert Nitske's book *The Life of Wilhelm Conrad Röntgen, Discoverer of the X Ray*: "In reality I had made several unexplainable observations which I carefully kept for future investigation, unfortunately not started in time, which must have been the effects of traces of wave radiation." For the rest of his life, Lenard dismissed Röntgen's claim as the discoverer of X-rays.

After "A New Kind of Rays" was published in the Physico-Medical Society's journal, Röntgen had several copies of the paper printed. On January 1, 1896, he sent them to leading physicists of the day, some of whom were his friends. To lend credibility to his writing, he sent several X-ray photographs along with the paper, including prints of the X-ray of Bertha's hand. Soon replies came flooding in, some congratulating Röntgen on his discovery, others exhibiting jealousy or even fear that he had unleashed some kind of new and deadly energy. Some simply could not believe what Röntgen had written. One professor from Berlin wrote, "I could not refrain from thinking that I was reading a fairy tale when I read the First Communication, but the name of the author and his sound proofs soon relieved me of any such delusion."[17]

It was, indeed, no delusion. His discovery was real, and was about to take the world by storm. For his efforts, in 1901 Wilhelm Conrad Röntgen would receive the first Nobel Prize ever awarded in the field of physics.

CHAPTER 3

X-rays in Medicine

Within days of the publication of Röntgen's paper, magazines and newspapers had picked up the story of the discovery of X-rays. Soon, people around the world were discussing Röntgen and his remarkable rays.

X-ray Mania

On January 7, 1896, a German newspaper called the *Frankfurter Zeitung* published an article, complete with X-ray photographs, about the future possibilities of Röntgen's X-rays:

> A Sensational Discovery: In the scientific circles of Vienna the news of a discovery, made by Professor of Physics Wilhelm Conrad Röntgen of Würzburg, is being discussed enthusiastically. If this discovery fulfills its promise, it constitutes an epoch-making result of research in exact science, which is destined to have interesting consequences along medical as well as physical lines. . . . A few examples of this sensational discovery are being circulated in scientific circles in Vienna and deservedly are creating great amazement. . . . Biologists and physicians, especially surgeons, will be very much interested in the practical uses of these rays, because they offer prospects of constituting a new and very valuable aid in diagnosis.[18]

But at this early stage in the development of X-rays, the excitement was not limited to the scientific and medical communities. Everyone, it seemed, wanted to learn more about X-rays, and experimenting with them became an international craze. The fact that the components needed to construct an X-ray machine could easily be obtained by just about anyone fueled the zeal of amateur X-ray experimenters. The world's first advertisement for X-ray equipment, a small classified notice, appeared in a Vienna newspaper on January 23, 1896—just a few weeks after Röntgen's First Communication was published. Other manufacturers were soon

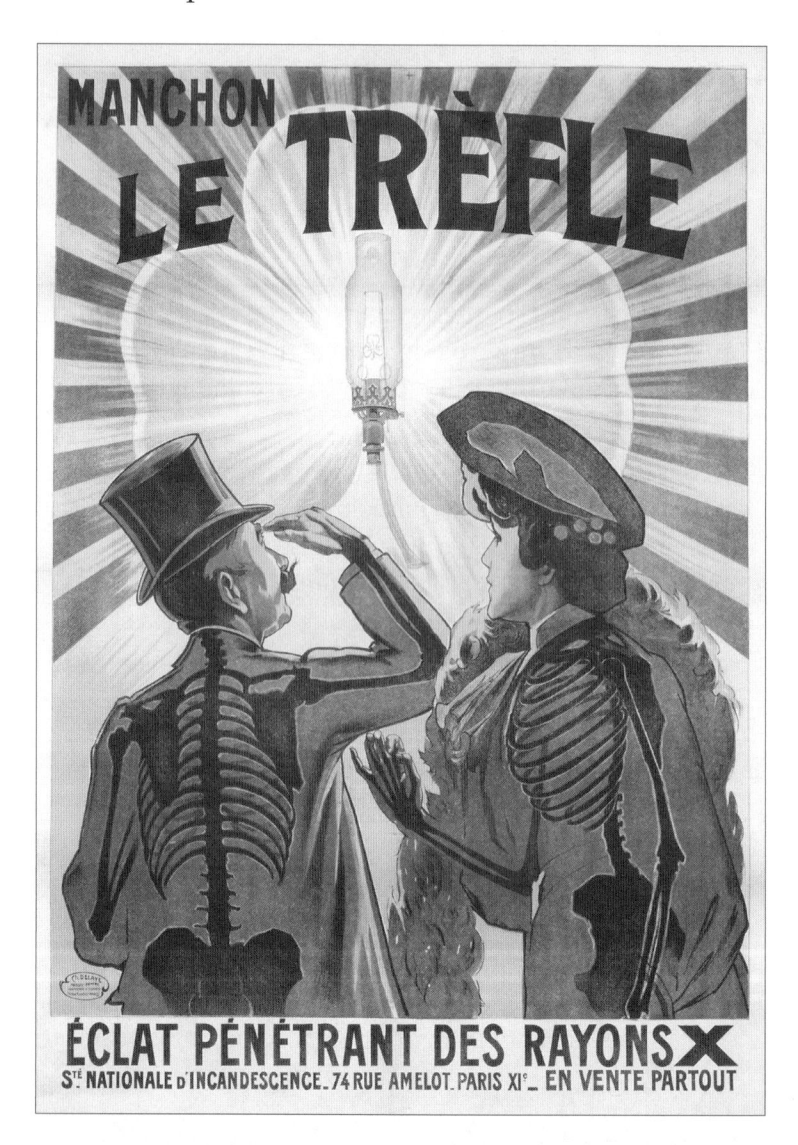

An early-twentieth-century French advertisement claims that this particular brand of gas lamps illuminates with the "penetrating brightness of X-rays."

touting their equipment with advertisements for X-ray tubes, high-voltage Ruhmkorff coils, and "absolutely indispensable" photographic plates that promised the "most gratifying success"[19] for both amateur experimenters and professional scientists and physicians.

As the X-ray fad spread, newspaper and magazine editors scrambled to find any story about X-rays to print. This resulted in the publication of many sensational articles and advertisements that either stretched the truth or were completely false. One article claimed that a medical school used X-rays to beam anatomical diagrams directly into students' brains. Another reported that an Iowa farmer used X-rays to transform a "cheap piece of metal worth about 13 cents to $153 worth of gold."[20] As X-rays were not yet well understood, readers had to rely on such stories for their information.

X-rays often were presented as an advancement in conventional photography. As the regular film camera photographed the exteriors of people and things, the new X-rays were said to be able to photograph the insides. In the late nineteenth century, modesty was valued in Victorian society, and the thought of an apparatus that could reveal a person's body under his or her clothing was alarming to many people. At least one London store began advertising X-ray–proof underwear. An ad in the United States offered X-ray opera glasses, small binoculars said to reveal everything of actors through their costumes while they performed on stage. Amazingly, a bill was introduced in the New Jersey legislature proposing a ban on X-ray opera glasses in the theater.

X-ray studios cropped up in many cities across the United States. These were not medical clinics run by doctors but rather commercial ventures set up by enterprising businessmen wanting to cash in on the X-ray craze. One advertisement for such a studio appeared on June 3, 1896: "Mr. M.F. Martin has opened an x-ray studio at 110 E. 26th St. in New York City, where pictures

> ## What's in a Name?
>
> Wilhelm Röntgen was adamant about not referring to X-rays as Röntgen rays. But there were many other names used to refer to X-rays in the early days of the technology. According to W. Robert Nitske in his book *The Life of Wilhelm Conrad Röntgen, Discoverer of the X Ray*, among them were:
>
> - electroskiagraphy
> - ixography
> - electrography
> - cathodography
> - fluorography
> - diagraphy
> - actinography
> - pyknoscopy
> - dark-light photography
> - tithonography
>
> With such tongue-twisting names proposed, it is fortunate that Röntgen's own simple term, X-rays, has become the standard used almost universally today.

of interior human structures will be taken. The consultation hours are from 1:00 to 2:00 and from 5:00 to 6:00. A lady assistant is in attendance."[21]

Some entrepreneurs even set up studios in their homes. It became fashionable to have "X-ray portraits" taken, not for any medical purpose but just for the novelty of owning such a unique item. The X-ray of a newly married woman's hand, for example, became a popular wedding souvenir. Department stores gave X-ray demonstrations, and coin-operated X-ray machines began appearing.

The widespread popularity of X-rays was due, in part, to the selflessness of Wilhelm Röntgen. After making his discovery, Röntgen refused to apply for a patent on X-rays. Had he done so, he could have made a fortune collecting licensing fees from anyone who wished to use his X-rays. But Röntgen felt that such important scientific discoveries should remain free for the benefit of all mankind and not just a source of profit for one man. He also resented the common practice in Europe to call X-rays "Röntgen rays," and he corrected such use whenever he could.

One thing Röntgen could not control was the public notoriety he was receiving due to the instant popularity of X-rays. He was inundated with constant requests to give lectures and demonstrate X-rays, and he could barely walk down the street without someone stopping him to offer congratulations on his discovery. All this attention upset Röntgen, for it kept him from continuing his experiments. He expressed his frustrations in a letter to a friend. "In a few days," Röntgen wrote, "I was disgusted with the whole thing. . . . Gradually I became accustomed to the uproar, but the storm [of publicity] cost time. For exactly four full weeks I have been unable to make a single experiment! Other people could work but not I. You have no idea how upset things were here."[22]

Thomas Edison's Fluoroscope

At the end of the nineteenth century, Thomas Alva Edison was America's foremost inventor. But not even he was immune to the excitement surrounding the remarkable new rays. Shortly after Röntgen's discovery, Edison built a darkroom at his New Jersey laboratory and began experimenting with X-rays. He searched for a chemical compound that would produce better results than the standard barium platinocyanide used on X-ray screens. The chemical he found was called calcium tungstate, and Edison used it to build a device he named a fluoroscope. The fluoroscope consisted of a tapered rectangular box with a screen coated with calcium tungstate at the large end. When the screen was aimed at an X-ray tube and a subject (usually the user's hand) was placed against the screen, an X-ray image could be viewed by looking into the fluoroscope's small end.

Not only did Edison's fluoroscope improve on the quality of similar devices created by other inventors, but he also brought X-rays to the attention of the general public. He arranged a demonstration of his fluoroscope at an electrical exhibition held in New York in May 1896. Thousands of curious people lined up to see the bones of their hands with a large fluoroscope Edison built especially for the exhibition. An article in the journal *Electrical Engineer* described the scene as people entered the darkened demonstration room:

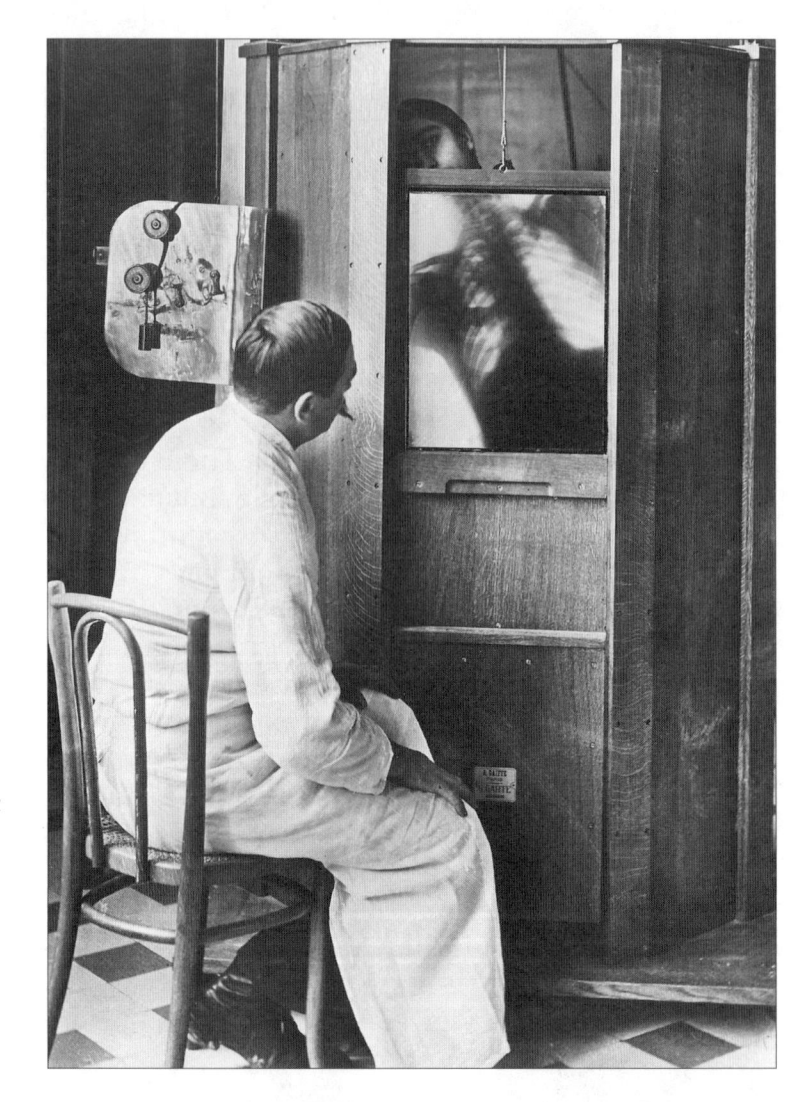

A doctor examines a patient's chest using a fluoroscope in this photo from the 1890s. Thomas Edison invented the fluoroscope in 1895 to improve the quality of X-ray images.

> On coming to the fluoroscope, the visitor was quietly told to slip his hand underneath the support and press it against the screen, palm side toward the eyes, and fingers close together. . . . Many of the visitors flinched as they got in front of the screen and refused to look, either at their own bones or anybody else's. Some crossed themselves devoutly after a fearsome glance, although, as a matter of fact, the great majority came out all smiles and laughter.[23]

Despite the success of Edison's demonstration, he abandoned his work with X-rays when his assistant, Clarence Dally, began showing signs that the X-rays seemed to have an adverse effect on the human body.

The First Medical X-rays

While the general public had become fascinated by X-rays as a curiosity, many physicians recognized that they could become a valuable diagnostic tool. An article in the January 30, 1896, edition of the magazine *Nation* describes the medical potential of X-rays:

> The importance of this discovery in its application to surgery as an aid to diagnosis in cases of disease or fracture of the bones is apparent. The [X-ray] photograph would reveal immediately and unmistakably the nature of the disorder without the long and often painful examination which the patient is now obliged to undergo.[24]

But while the potential for X-rays seemed unlimited, the medical community was slow to adopt this new technology. Perhaps unsure if the X-ray fad would last, and somewhat settled in their ways, many doctors only used X-rays as a last resort when all other diagnostic methods had been tried. Still, some physicians, many of them at university medical schools, enthusiastically embraced X-rays and used them in their medical practices.

The first clinical X-ray photograph taken in the United States was made on February 3, 1896. Edwin B. Frost, a physics professor at Dartmouth College in New Hampshire, made the X-ray image for his brother

Gilman Frost, a doctor. The patient, fourteen-year-old Eddie McCarthy, had fallen while ice skating and complained of pain in his left wrist. Frost x-rayed the boy's arm in the physics lab at Dartmouth, and upon developing the plate, he confirmed that the wrist was, indeed, broken. Of the procedure, Frost wrote, "It was possible yesterday to test the method on a broken arm. After an exposure of 20 minutes, the plate on development showed the fracture in the ulna very distinctively. Comment upon the numerous applications of the new method in the sciences and arts would be superfluous."[25]

Another famous early X-ray photograph, made by Michael Pupin of Columbia University in New York, demonstrated the ability of X-rays to reveal foreign objects in the body. Prescott Butler, a New York lawyer, had been accidentally shot with a shotgun, leaving some three dozen pellets lodged in his hand. Pupin x-rayed Butler's hand on February 14, 1896, and the resulting photograph clearly showed the lead pellets as bright white dots against the bones in Butler's hand. The surgeon, William Bull, could then remove the pellets without having to do painful probing of the wounds to locate them. The remarkably clear X-ray was widely published in newspapers and magazines. Years later, Pupin sent a copy of the X-ray to the chairman of the Historical Roentgen Committee in Chicago, describing the photograph as "the first X-ray picture to guide a surgical operation in the United States."[26]

Dangerous Rays

With all the excitement over the amazing capabilities of X-rays, one aspect went unrecognized for a time: the fact that X-rays could be dangerous or even lethal. In the early experimental stage, no one had any idea of the hazards of X-rays. Early tubes sent X-rays in all directions, not just toward the photographic plate recording the image. Doctors routinely exposed their patients to prolonged doses of X-rays (sometimes for an hour or

> ### America's First Radiologist
>
> In the beginning, medical interest in X-rays was widespread among all kinds of doctors. But it was not long before some physicians decided to become radiologists, specializing in taking and interpreting X-rays. Francis Henry Williams of Boston has been called America's first radiologist.
>
> Born in Boston in 1852, Williams studied engineering at the Massachusetts Institute of Technology before receiving his medical degree. This technical training allowed Williams to understand X-rays better than many doctors of his time. As a result, he was able to introduce many advancements that made radiology safer and more accurate for both doctors and patients. Williams advocated the use of a metal diaphragm on X-ray tubes to focus the beam for a sharper image and to protect the patient from stray radiation. Because of the precautions he took, he never suffered the X-ray–related illnesses experienced by so many other early X-ray workers.
>
> Williams once demonstrated the value of fluoroscopy by drawing the outline of a patient's enlarged heart on his chest using the old-fashioned percussion method. He then observed the heart with a fluoroscope; the image of the heart on the fluorescent screen matched the drawn outline almost exactly.
>
> During his years of practice, Williams x-rayed more than 150,000 patients. He also wrote the first radiology textbook, titled *The Roentgen Rays in Medicine and Surgery*, which became widely read by medical students.

more) without any kind of protection, either for the patients or for themselves. The first sign of danger was usually dermatitis, an inflammation or reddening of the skin similar to a sunburn. One doctor recalled:

> The prescription of dosage was so uncertain and the results apparently so capricious that all one could really do was to place the patient under the machine and hope for the best. Patients were burned from unexpected leaks, and on one or more occasions, it is said, actually electrocuted on the treatment table.[27]

There was another side effect of X-rays. People who had had X-rays taken began reporting that their hair was falling out in the areas where the X-ray beams had been applied. The effect was not permanent, however, and several months later the hair would grow back. Some newspapers wrote amusing articles about this phenomenon, quipping that men could soon stop shaving and instead simply x-ray their beards away.

An X-ray technician from the early twentieth century wears a heavy lead apron and goggles. Most early X-ray workers did not wear protection and many developed cancer.

But the adverse effects of X-rays were no laughing matter. Most researchers x-rayed their hands every day to make sure their machines were working. After many months of such exposure, the resulting dermatitis could progress to a more dangerous disease, skin cancer. If allowed to spread throughout the body, the effects of this cancer could be lethal. At the time, the only way to prevent this spread was to cut off the affected limb.

Amputated fingers, hands, and arms became commonplace among X-ray workers. Even then, this drastic measure sometimes came too late.

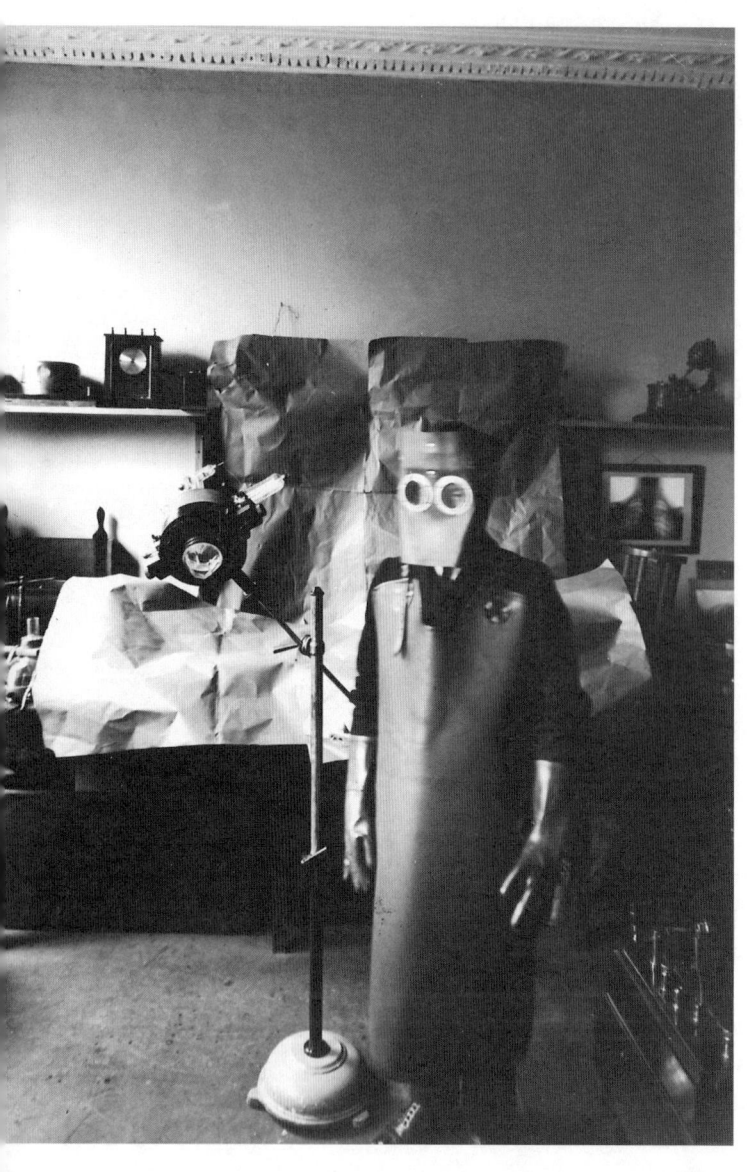

Clarence Dally, Thomas Edison's assistant, became the first American X-ray fatality, succumbing to X-ray–induced cancer in 1904. Because the harmful effects of X-rays often occurred at some length after exposure, many people failed to make the connection between the two. And many doctors downplayed the danger for fear of scaring off patients. "The x-ray," commented one physician, "... is incapable of injuring the tissues of the patients, and their dermatitis, which has been called an x-ray 'burn,' is the result of an interference with the nutrition of the part by the induced static charges."[28] But physicians and X-ray equipment manufacturers could not avoid the truth for long, and soon steps were being taken to protect both the doctors and their patients.

Since lead blocks X-rays, manufacturers began putting lead shields around their tubes to limit stray X-rays. Lead-lined protective suits, consisting of a lead apron, long gloves, a hood, and goggles, were cumbersome and odd-looking, but they protected the wearer from X-rays. Eventually, doctors began carrying small pieces of unexposed film with them when taking X-rays. Upon being developed, a film that was fogged indicated exposure to X-rays, allowing the doctor to limit further exposure. These films were the forerunners of modern-day film badges, called dosimeters, which consist of a small piece of photographic film encased in plastic and clipped to clothing. Worn by X-ray technicians, film badges detect stray X-rays and, when developed, indicate if a person has received a harmful dosage of radiation. International conferences on radiation were held in 1925 and 1928 to develop definitions for units of radiation. Fittingly, the unit of X-radiation was called the roentgen. In 1931 the maximum allowable daily exposure to radiation, called the "tolerance dose," was established at .01 roentgen.

Advances in Radiology

Early X-rays were limited to recording images of solid objects that easily blocked the path of the X-ray beam: bones, bullets, needles, shrapnel, and other solid objects inside the body, either naturally or by accident. But physicians wanted a way to observe other body structures that were made of soft tissues rather than solid bones. In Vienna, Austria, two doctors had the idea of injecting into the body a material that would block X-rays. Such a material, they reasoned, might reveal the soft tissues and other structures not ordinarily seen in X-rays. Unable to find a willing patient to experiment on, the doctors injected a hand from a cadaver with a fluid that contained calcium, a compound found in human bones. Since bones blocked X-rays, they contended, calcium elsewhere in the body should do the same. They were right; when filled with the calcium solution, the veins in the hand clearly showed up on an X-ray. This was the first angiogram, an X-ray of the blood vessels, and the injected liquid became known as a contrast medium. Soon researchers developed contrast media that were safe for use on live patients, including liquids that could be swallowed or otherwise introduced into body cavities. Walter Dandy, a surgeon at Johns Hopkins Hospital in Baltimore, Maryland, discovered that air was a good contrast medium, and he used it to make X-rays of the brain (encephalograms). Other contrast media, including lipiodol (an oil mixed with iodine), sodium iodide, and barium, were used to reveal other parts of the body, including the esophagus, stomach, and intestines.

X-rays have been used to identify other soft tissue diseases. Tuberculosis, an infectious disease of the lungs, has plagued humankind since ancient times. Diagnosing this disease had been mainly done by listening to the lungs with a stethoscope. While taking X-rays to diagnose broken ribs, Lewis Cole, a New York doctor, sometimes noticed shadows in a patient's lungs. He wondered if these shadows were caused by tuberculosis. Despite skepticism from colleagues, Cole performed experiments on the tubercular lungs of cadavers, and he ultimately proved that X-rays could be used to diagnose tuberculosis. As tuberculosis is a highly contagious disease, early diagnosis is important. By using X-rays, doctors could promptly admit tuberculosis patients to sanitariums (resort-type facilities for chronically ill patients) for treatment and isolation before the disease had a chance to spread.

In the decade after Röntgen's discovery, manufacturers of X-ray equipment began improving their products, creating better X-ray tubes and more reliable power supplies. Exposure times became shorter, meaning less risk to patients and doctors alike. In 1913 a physicist named

William Coolidge developed a new kind of tube, called a hot cathode tube. This tube produced clearer X-rays, could be adjusted for high or low penetration of the body, and was safer because it produced less scattered X-rays. Due to the adjustable nature of the X-rays produced by this new tube, radiologists could replace several ordinary tubes with just one Coolidge tube. Modern X-ray tubes are of essentially the same design as Coolidge's original tube. By 1918 the fragile glass photographic plates that all X-rays had previously been made on were gradually being replaced by lightweight, flexible film, similar to the X-rays we are familiar with today.

X-ray equipment manufacturers sent trained salesmen on the road to market their improved X-ray machines to doctors and hospitals throughout the United States. As early as 1910 a survey showed that two-thirds of American hospitals owned X-ray machines; by the end of the 1920s, X-rays had become a standard part of medical procedure. As X-ray machines became increasingly monopolized by the medical field (and more expensive as well), non-medical users of X-rays, such as photographers, began closing up their commercial X-ray studios. The period of X-rays as a popular fad was over, but the era of X-rays as a serious medical tool was just beginning.

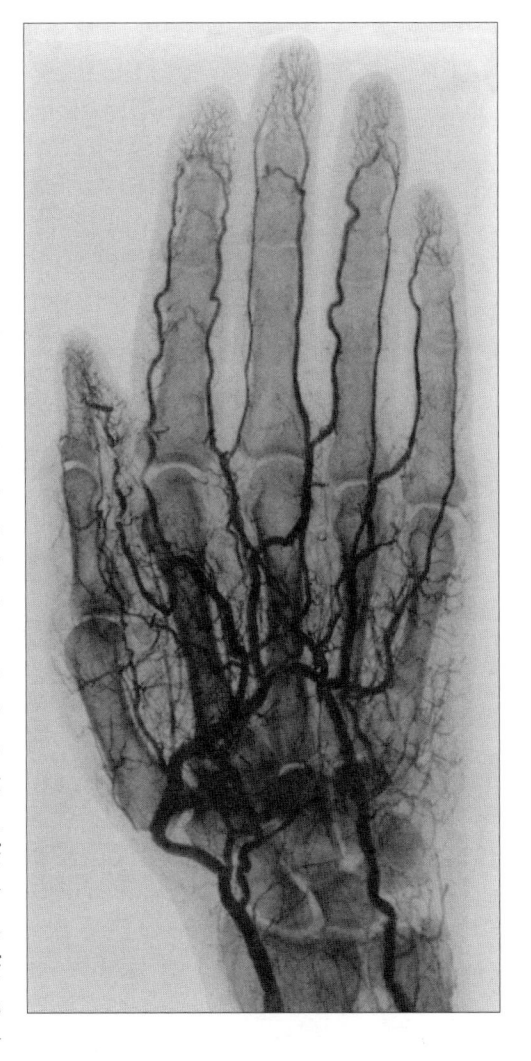

An Australian doctor made this angiogram of the blood vessels in a cadaver's hand in 1904.

X-rays in War and Peace

The advantages of X-rays were especially suited to military medical practice, where bullets lodged in bodies, embedded shrapnel, and shattered bones were common battlefield injuries. British military hospitals had installed X-ray machines as early as 1896. Portable X-ray units were used in field hospitals near battle zones, with the electricity to run the machines provided by soldiers pedaling specially modified bicycles. During World War I the French converted twenty automobiles into mobile X-ray units. These vehicles brought X-ray machines to the front lines to help military doctors as they operated on wounded soldiers. Women were trained to assist physicians in the operation of these mobile stations, but the women often were able to run their units independently. In addition to these mobile X-ray units, some two hundred stationary X-ray facilities were also established.

When the United States entered World War I in 1917, many civilian doctors who had been using X-rays in their practices joined the U.S. Army Medical Corps. In addition, schools were established in many U.S. cities to teach the use of X-ray machines to physicians with no prior experience with the new technology. These doctors served throughout Europe during the war, and after the hostilities ended, they came home with new knowledge and a new appreciation for the value of X-rays in clinical diagnosis. Even army physicians who had not considered the advantages of X-rays before were often persuaded, through their war experiences, to utilize X-rays in their own private practices after the war.

The acceptance of X-rays as a routine method of diagnosis for patients in civilian hospitals came more slowly. Despite the X-ray's obvious potential, many physicians were set in their ways. They were not convinced that X-rays added any useful information about an injury or illness that could not be obtained by more traditional means. The physical examination remained the doctor's primary diagnostic tool. One study of X-rays concluded that "no one will for a moment suppose that the vacuum tube and induction coil will, or ever can, displace the sense of touch guided by a well-balanced and experienced mind."[29]

X-rays in Medicine

Another advance in the history of X-rays was tomography, or taking an X-ray of a slice of the human body. In the 1920s a man named Jean Kieffer (coincidentally, a tuberculosis patient) had the idea that by introducing motion into the X-ray process, parts of a patient's body normally blocked by bones might be x-rayed. In tomography, the X-ray tube and the film were placed on opposite sides of the patient and were focused on the area to be examined. Then the tube and film were rotated around the patient, and the resulting X-ray revealed a "slice" of the patient, with obstructions (such as bones) blurred out due to the motion of the apparatus. The tube and film assembly could be moved vertically to X-ray different slices of the patient, and the thickness of each slice could be adjusted as well. A sequence of tomographs could be created to represent an organ or other part of the body not visible to normal X-rays. Other researchers came up with designs for a tomograph machine, including one that moved

A soldier lies still as an X-ray of his skull is taken at a military hospital during World War I. Military doctors made wide use of X-ray technology throughout the war.

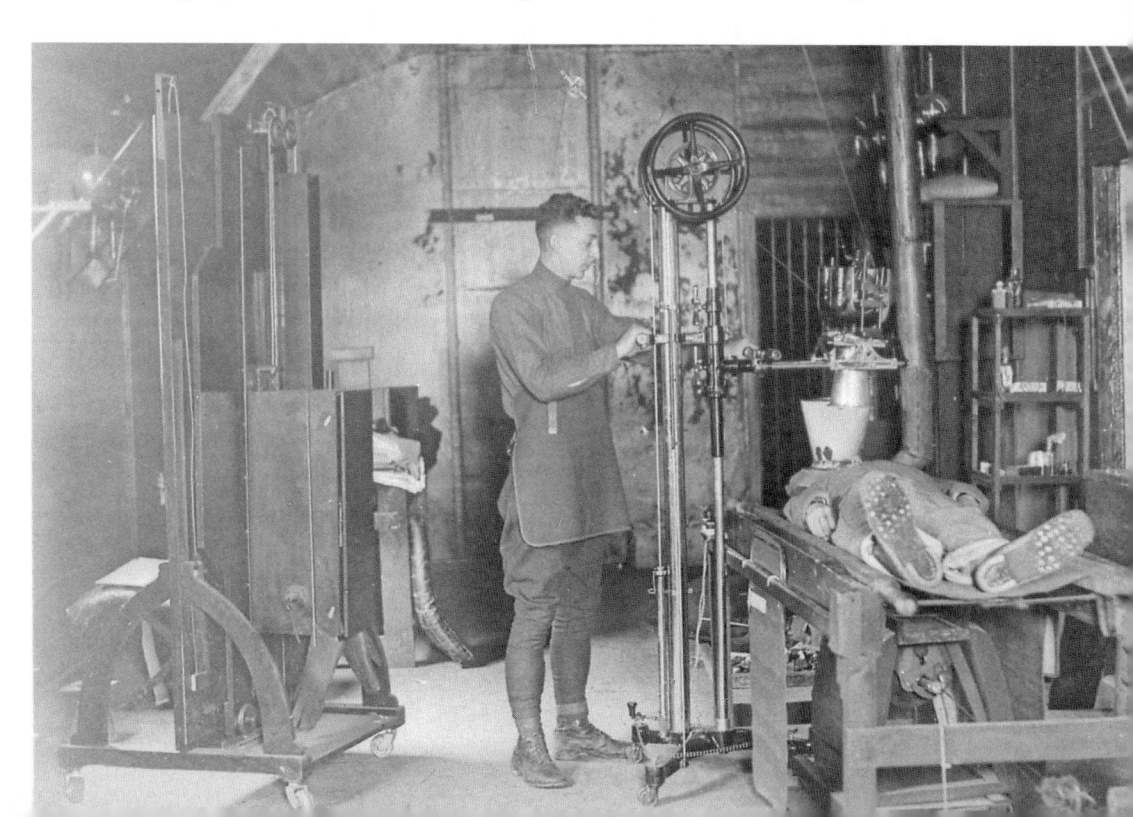

> ### Fitting Shoes with X-rays
>
> From the 1920s until about the mid-twentieth century, hospitals and clinics were not the only places one could find X-ray machines. A trip to the local shoe store allowed anyone to take a look at the bones in their feet with a device called a shoe-fitting fluoroscope.
>
> The device was housed in a large wooden cabinet, with a raised platform in front and an opening into which the feet were placed. On top of the cabinet, eyepieces allowed the customer and the shoe salesman to view the interior. When the fluoroscope was turned on, a ghostly greenish image of the bones in the feet could be seen, ostensibly allowing the salesman to observe the foot structure and thus choose the proper shoe. Children were delighted to see their bones, and adults were impressed with this unique use of technology. By the 1950s some ten thousand machines were in use.
>
> Soon, however, people became concerned about the effects of excess radiation, a fear based partly on the growing nuclear weapons arsenals of the United States and the Soviet Union. If radioactive fallout was dangerous, many reasoned, perhaps the use of radiation-generating devices like the shoe-fitting fluoroscope should be limited. This attitude gradually prevailed, and by the 1960s most of the shoe-fitting fluoroscopes had been removed from stores.

the patient's body while the X-ray tube and film remained stationary. But the inventors could not find a market for their machine: manufacturers doubted that it really worked, and doctors complained that the quality of tomographs was poorer than ordinary X-rays. By the 1930s, however, the quality of tomographs was beginning to improve. In St. Louis, a hospital installed a machine based on Kieffer's design, and by 1939 over one thousand tomographs had been taken. Other hospitals across the country took note, and soon the market for Kieffer's machine was booming.

As essential as X-rays were becoming for diagnosing a variety of diseases, some doctors were using the new rays for another purpose: to actually treat illnesses.

Chapter 4

Therapeutic Uses of X-rays

With the steady increase in cases of X-ray burns and scarring that sometimes led to disfiguring amputations, doctors soon realized that these new rays could be harmful, even lethal, to themselves and their patients. But they also began to consider that, if X-rays could have such damaging effects on human tissues, perhaps if properly controlled these same rays might actually have a healing effect on certain diseases. There was as yet no scientific evidence that would confirm this theory, but many physicians were curious. In the spirit of entrepreneurship that had brought X-rays to the public in such a short time, they began experimenting with the therapeutic uses of X-rays.

Healing the Skin

Using light as a therapeutic agent can be traced as far back as ancient Egypt and Greece. Physicians there erected temples where their patients could benefit from the healing characteristics of sunlight. They knew that exposure to the sun improved their patients' conditions, even if they did not understand that sunlight strengthened the immune system, hastened the repair of damaged cells, and relieved pain. In Röntgen's time, physicians were experimenting with light as a germicidal, or germ-killing, agent. It was known that light (actually invisible ultraviolet light) could kill bacteria.

Given this germicidal quality of light, it was reasoned that perhaps the new kind of light, X-rays, might have the same effect. Although numerous experiments in killing germs with X-rays were made, none was successful. Even so, later clinical experience showed X-rays to be effective in treating certain infectious diseases.

In the late nineteenth century, a Danish physician, Neils Finsen, experimented with light for treating skin conditions. He was interested in the effects of light on humans, especially ultraviolet light (which might more accurately be called ultraviolet rays). Ultraviolet (UV) light is produced by the sun and some artificial light

The Electromagnetic Spectrum

Visible light, X-rays, radio waves, and gamma rays are all parts of a continuous band of radiant energy known as the electromagnetic (EM) spectrum. Scientists have categorized different kinds of EM energy based on their wavelengths—the distance between the peaks of a radiant energy source's waves. The different types of EM waves are also classified by their energy and frequency. Wavelength, energy, and frequency are all related to each other mathematically.

The EM spectrum runs from radio waves at the low end (longest wavelength, lowest energy) to gamma rays at the high end (shortest wavelength, highest energy). In between are visible light waves that allow people to see, invisible light (such as ultraviolet light) that can produce a healthy tan or a painful sunburn, radar waves for tracking aircraft, and microwaves that can cook your dinner. X-rays, having relatively short wavelengths, fall just below high-energy gamma rays in the electromagnetic spectrum.

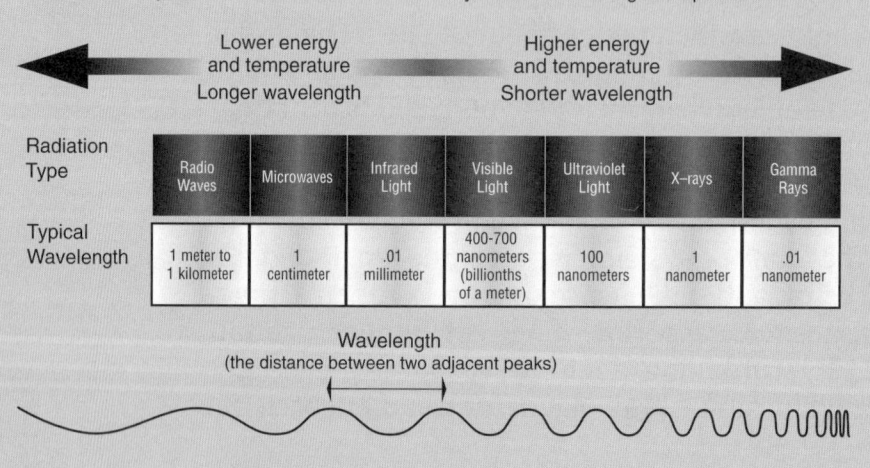

⬅ Lower energy and temperature / Longer wavelength

Higher energy and temperature / Shorter wavelength ➡

Radiation Type	Radio Waves	Microwaves	Infrared Light	Visible Light	Ultraviolet Light	X-rays	Gamma Rays
Typical Wavelength	1 meter to 1 kilometer	1 centimeter	.01 millimeter	400-700 nanometers (billionths of a meter)	100 nanometers	1 nanometer	.01 nanometer

Wavelength
(the distance between two adjacent peaks)

sources. It is invisible to us because it falls outside the spectrum of light we can see. The positive germ-killing effects of ultraviolet light are well known. But other, less beneficial effects can be all too apparent: It is the UV rays from the sun that cause painful and sometimes dangerous sunburn. Finsen discovered that applying light helped patients suffering from various skin diseases, such as lupus vulgaris, a disfiguring disease also known as skin tuberculosis. For his work, Finsen was awarded a Nobel Prize in 1903, two years after Röntgen had received his Nobel Prize for X-rays. Light therapy remained a popular form of treatment until antibiotics were developed to treat skin diseases more effectively.

Finsen's light therapy sometimes caused a reddening of his patients' skin, the same way that X-rays often did. In addition, X-rays are very close to ultraviolet rays in the electromagnetic spectrum. This led doctors to speculate that X-rays might also be used to combat skin diseases the way UV rays were. In 1898 two doctors in Austria used X-rays to successfully treat lupus vulgaris in several patients. In the United States, a San Francisco physician named Philip Mills Jones also had success with the use of X-rays on a patient who had lupus lesions on his forehead. Jones later described his method of treatment.

> There were present three ulcerating points and one large, hard nodule which had not yet broken down. A sheet of lead was arranged so as to protect the whole of the head save the lupus area; a hole cut in the lead sheet allowed the x-rays to reach all the diseased areas, with the exception of one of the ulcerating points. This one small point was protected as a sort of control upon the treatment. . . . At the end of four weeks the whole area, with the exception of the one ulcer protected, was healed and the nodule had disappeared.[30]

Some physicians discovered the therapeutic value of X-rays by accident while treating patients for other conditions. For example, a doctor who was using X-rays to remove unwanted hair from a female patient noticed that acne on her chin and around her mouth had cleared up after the X-ray treatments. Based on this clinical evidence, the doctor treated acne in thirteen other patients. X-rays were also found to be useful in treating other skin conditions, such as eczema and ringworm of the scalp. While these are not life-threatening conditions, they can be very noticeable and embarrassing to those who suffer from them. Before X-rays were found to be harmful to living tissue, they were used to alleviate these conditions. But their use declined as the dangerous nature of X-rays became known and as other treatments, such as antibiotics and lasers, were developed to treat the same conditions more safely and effectively.

X-ray therapy did, however, bring new treatment to another, more dangerous, form of skin disease: cancer.

Combating Cancer

In an article published in the *Philadelphia Medical Journal* in 1900, two doctors wrote, "There is no disease physicians like less to encounter than carcinoma [cancer] in any of its forms."[31] In the early days of X-ray therapy, it was natural for physicians to want to test the new technology on one of humankind's most dreaded diseases. The first type of cancer X-ray therapy was tried on the most noticeable, and often the easiest to treat, form of the disease, skin cancer.

In the early years of building X-ray machines, it was found that the best rays for diagnostic use were generated by tubes that had not been completely evacuated. That is, these so-called soft vacuum tubes did not contain total vacuums because some air was left inside. But as they were used, the vacuums in these tubes gradually increased, resulting in "hard" tubes that limited the amount of the desirable X-rays they emitted. But the rays that remained were found to be higher energy rays, which were most suitable for therapeutic uses. So, many older hard tubes, rather than being discarded or returned to the factory for rebuilding, found a new life in treating cancer and other diseases. Manufacturers soon began making hard tubes specifically for X-ray therapy.

Thor Stenbeck, a Swedish doctor often referred to as Sweden's first radiologist, was probably the first physician to use X-rays to treat skin cancer. Cancer is a disease in which normally healthy cells begin to multiply out of control. If this growth is not halted, the cancer cells can spread throughout the body and attack healthy cells, often resulting in death. Stenbeck knew that X-rays could harm healthy cells, causing radiation burns on the skin. Might X-rays likewise damage, or possibly even destroy, cancer cells? He discovered that X-rays inflict damage on abnormal cancer cells more than they harm normal, healthy cells. Stenbeck used high-energy X-rays to destroy the multiplying skin cancer cells and thus cured the disease.

X-ray therapy soon became a standard tool for dermatologists, but other physicians also were experimenting with the rays on types of cancer that were more difficult to treat.

Emil Grubbé, a Chicago physician, claimed to be the first to use X-rays in fighting breast cancer, in January

Dr. Skinner's Case

The first years of the twentieth century saw a boom in the number of doctors experimenting with X-rays for therapeutic uses. One of the most famous early cases of curing illness with X-rays involved a doctor named Clarence E. Skinner.

His patient was a thirty-nine-year-old teacher who, in 1898, had undergone surgery for what was thought to be a benign (noncancerous) abdominal tumor. The growth returned, however, and was found to be cancerous. When traditional treatments failed and the patient's condition was considered hopeless, she was referred to Skinner.

In 1902 Skinner began X-ray treatments, and over the next several months administered forty-six X-ray therapy sessions. The tumor began to shrink, and soon the patient was able to return to teaching—something she had not been able to do for more than a year.

Here was an early case of cancer that, once considered hopeless, was cured by X-ray therapy. Five years after her final X-ray treatment, Skinner's patient was still free of cancer, although she did suffer from X-ray burns.

1896. According to Grubbé's own account, his patient, Rose Lee, was "placed on her back on an improvised operating table and made as comfortable as could be."[32] He used lead sheets to protect her during the treatment, which consisted of one hour of X-rays administered daily. Over the next several weeks, Grubbé gave his patient eighteen X-ray treatments. Unfortunately, the cancer was already too far advanced, and Lee died within a month. Nevertheless, Grubbé was not shy about establishing his place in the annals of X-ray therapy, writing that, "for the first time in history, X rays had been used for *treatments*, not diagnostic purposes. . . . That was the beginning of the treatment of diseases with X rays; that was the origin of X ray therapy."[33] In addition, Grubbé claimed to be the first person to suffer injuries due to X-rays. Not all historians accept Grubbé's accounts as truthful. Other physicians at the time were also beginning the experimental use of X-rays to treat serious forms of cancer. One thing that is not disputed is that Emil Grubbé was one of the many pioneers to lose his life to X-rays. Throughout his lifetime he endured no less than eighty-three operations to relieve the disfiguring effects of X-rays on his face and left arm. He died in 1960 of X-ray–induced cancer, thus fulfilling his prediction that, "I, too, will die a victim of natural science, a martyr to the X ray."[34]

Doctors and scientists knew that X-rays could be a powerful tool in fighting disease. This knowledge led to other types of radiation being used for therapeutic purposes. One such form of radiation, called radium, came from an element which was discovered by a young Polish woman studying at a university in France.

Marie Curie's Radium

Marya Sklodowska was born on November 7, 1867, in Warsaw, Poland. A brilliant student in high school, she eventually entered the Sorbonne, a famous university in Paris. Now calling herself Marie, the French version of her Polish name, she pursued scientific studies in

Therapeutic Uses of X-rays 63

such subjects as physics, mathematics, and chemistry. She married a thirty-five-year-old scientist named Pierre Curie in 1895, the same year that Wilhelm Röntgen discovered X-rays. As with many scientists of that day, Röntgen's discovery aroused the Curies' interest in radiation. Marie decided to investigate radiation as her university research project.

Marie's work centered on a previous discovery made by physicist Antoine-Henri Becquerel, who found that an element called uranium gave off rays similar to X-rays. Becquerel eventually lost interest in these rays, but Marie continued studying them. She also coined the term *radioactive* to describe material that emitted

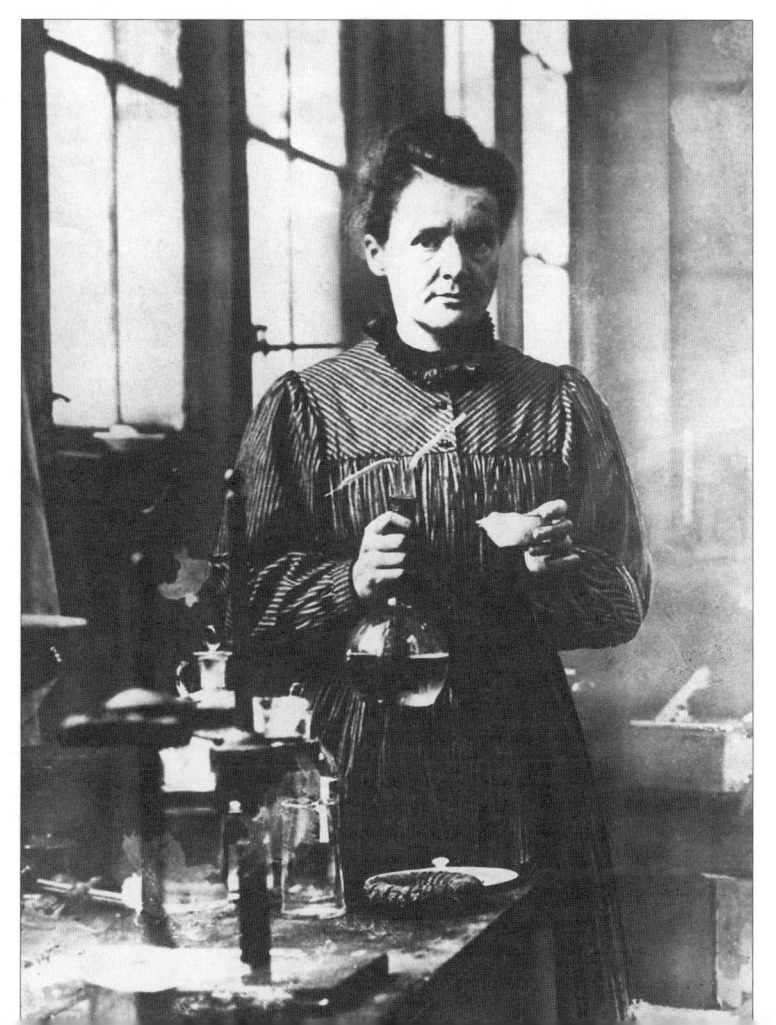

Polish physicist Marie Curie won two Nobel Prizes for her groundbreaking research with radioactive materials, which emit rays similar to X-rays.

rays. Working with pitchblende, or uranium ore, Marie and Pierre discovered two new sources of strong radiation: polonium, named for Marie's homeland, and radium, a source of radiation even stronger than uranium. It was a difficult task, as Marie explained some years later:

> I thought that there should be in the minerals some unknown element having a much greater radioactivity than uranium.... I wanted to find and to separate that element, and I settled to that work with Professor Curie. We thought it would be done in several weeks or months, but it was not so. It took many years of hard work to finish that task. There was not one new element, there were several of them. But the most important is radium, which could be separated in a pure state.
>
> Now the special interest of radium is in the intensity of its rays, which [are] several million times greater than the uranium rays. And the effects of the rays make the radium important. If we take a practical point of view, the most important property of the rays is the production of physiological effects on the cells of the human organism. These effects may be used for the cure of several diseases. Good results have been obtained in many cases. What is considered particularly important is the treatment of cancer.[35]

By 1913 radium was being used to treat certain types of cancer. Marie Curie won two Nobel Prizes for her work with radium, the only person to be awarded a Nobel Prize in both chemistry and physics. Unfortunately, like many of the X-ray pioneers, Curie was physically affected by a lifetime of accumulated exposure to radiation: She died of leukemia in 1934.

Targeting Cancer

Radiation can be administered to a cancer patient in a variety of ways. Depending on the type of cancer and its location in the body, doctors may decide to use X-rays or other forms of radiation to destroy the cancer cells. Radiation therapy (also known as radiotherapy) can be used either alone or in addition to surgery. Surgery is often used to remove a tumor, which is a mass of cancerous cells, ideally before the cancer has a chance to spread. But a tumor may be located in a part of the body where surgery would be dangerous or impossible to perform. In these instances, radiation can be used to attack the tumor. Sometimes a tumor may be too large to be successfully removed by surgery. In these cases, radiation can be employed to shrink the tumor, destroying it completely or reducing its size so that it can be safely removed by a surgeon. There are two types of radiotherapy used in modern medicine: external and internal. These designations refer to the location of the source of the radiation used in the treatment, which may be either outside the body or within the body itself.

External radiotherapy most commonly employs a large machine called a linear accelerator. Doctors knew that high-energy X-rays produced by "hard" X-ray tubes were the most efficient for killing cancer cells. It was reasonable to assume, then, that these X-rays would work even better if they had even more energy. Physicists use huge devices called particle accelerators to study the inner workings of the atom. These accelerators use magnetic fields to increase the energy of tiny particles of matter, speeding them up to velocities near the speed of light. Some accelerators send the particles spinning around a circular track to increase their speed; others, called linear accelerators (linacs), move the particles in a straight line. When a high enough speed is reached, the high-energy particle is directed toward a target, either a stationary object or another particle moving in the opposite direction. When the two collide, an atom is freed from the target and is broken down into smaller components for scientists to study. Particle accelerators are sometimes referred to as atom smashers for this violent, energy-releasing collision.

Linear accelerators in the medical field produce high-energy X-rays or other types of radiation (particularly gamma rays, which are close to X-rays in the electromagnetic spectrum) that can effectively treat many kinds of cancerous tumors. The X-rays produced by these machines are far stronger than X-rays used for imaging purposes. Linear accelerators are usually located in a room of a hospital or clinic that is shielded against radiation leakage. Although the typical linac is very large and heavy, weighing up to several tons, it is designed so that the operator can move it with great precision to aim the radiation beam at the precise point on the patient's body. Using microwave technology, the linear accelerator speeds up a stream of electrons, which are aimed at a metal target. When impact occurs, X-rays are produced by the target and directed at the tumor and away from the surrounding healthy tissue. Treatments are not given all at once; instead, they are administered over an extended period of time, with patients receiving daily doses over several weeks or months.

A Dangerous Treatment

What do children, pilots, scuba divers, and submarine crews have in common? Beginning in the 1940s, many members of these groups were treated with radium for inner ear problems. Known as nasopharyngeal radium irradiation (NRI), this therapy, according to the National Cancer Institute Web site, involved,

inserting two cylinders of radioactive radium sulfate through the nostrils into the nasopharyngeal opening (the space behind the nose and mouth) for short lengths of time. Typically, each cylinder contained 25 milligrams of radium sulfate, and patients were exposed for three sessions of 8.5 minutes each.

Using radium to shrink the lymph tissue in the throat was thought to alleviate ear infections in children. Military doctors commonly used NRI to relieve ear pain in pilots, divers, and submariners. What doctors did not take into account was the proximity of delicate structures, such as the brain and the thyroid and pituitary glands, which might be damaged by the radiation. Concerned with the long-term effects of radium on these organs, physicians finally ended NRI treatments in the 1970s.

The ability to focus the X-ray beam on just the tumor is one of the main benefits of radiotherapy using the linear accelerator. Other advantages include reduced treatment times, the ability to penetrate even deep-seated tumors, and the fact that it is a less invasive procedure than surgery. It is frequently the treatment of choice for tumors that are localized—that is, tumors that have not invaded nearby healthy tissue or spread to other parts of the body. Even in cases where the cancer has spread, X-ray radiotherapy can be useful in relieving pain associated with advanced cancer. Radiation therapy is also often used after a tumor has been surgically removed, killing any cancer cells left behind after the surgery.

Stereotactic radiosurgery is an extremely precise form of radiation therapy used primarily for treating brain tumors. Despite the name, this procedure is not traditional, invasive surgery. Instead, it uses several beams of high-intensity radiation focused on the exact spot of the brain tumor. In brain surgery it is especially important to protect the healthy tissue surrounding the tumor. During stereotactic radiosurgery, the patient's head is placed in a helmet or head frame that immobilizes it, so that the radiation beams stay focused on the tumor.

The procedure is performed with either a linear accelerator or a device known as a Gamma Knife. The Gamma Knife uses radiation produced by the isotope cobalt 60 to attack the brain tumor. The "blades" of the Gamma Knife are actually 201 streams of gamma radiation aimed directly at the tumor. Individually, these radiation streams are relatively weak. But at their focal point in the tumor, they are strong enough to destroy the cancer cells and shrink the tumor. This type of procedure avoids the risks of infection and bleeding inherent in traditional brain surgery. It is also virtually painless, except for some minor discomfort caused by the helmet. And since it is usually performed on an outpatient basis, operating room and recovery room costs are eliminated.

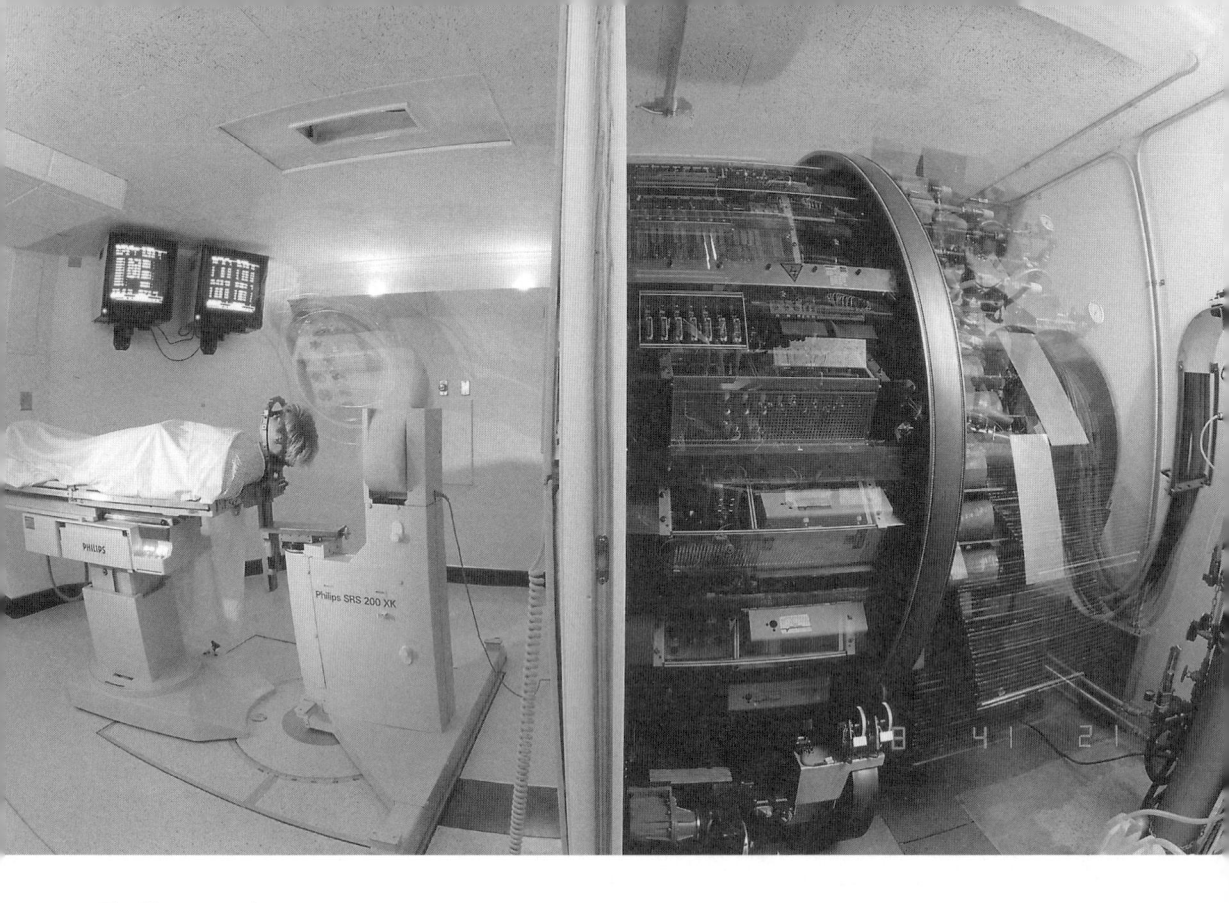

The linear accelerator behind the wall on the right produces high-energy radiation that targets brain tumors growing in the patient lying on the treatment table on the left.

Similar to stereotactic radiosurgery is stereotactic radiotherapy. This procedure uses smaller doses, called fractionated radiation (administered over several days or weeks) or hyperfractionated radiation (given several times a day), rather than a single larger dose. The frame to hold the patient steady during stereotactic radiotherapy is usually attached to the machine rather than to the patient's head. Daily treatments may last several weeks, but, as with radiosurgery, there are fewer side effects than with traditional brain surgery.

Attacking Cancer from Within

Standard X-ray therapy attacks cancer cells by beaming radiation to a tumor from outside the body. Internal radiation therapy fights cancer by placing a source of radiation in the patient's body or in a body cavity near the site of the tumor. This type of treatment is also called brachytherapy ("short therapy"), which refers to the short distances the radiation travels within the body. With internal radiotherapy, the radiation is supplied by

Therapeutic Uses of X-rays

a radioactive material placed in the patient's body, either within the tumor or as close to it as possible. This material, often called cobalt 60, decays at a steady rate, continuously emitting gamma rays. These rays act like X-rays to kill cancer cells.

In some types of cancer, the radiation source can be introduced into body cavities near the site of the tumor. For example, in cases of cervical cancer, the radioactive source is placed into the vagina, where it can attack the tumor without the need for surgery. To treat other types of tumors, such as prostate cancer, radioactive pellets or "seeds" are surgically implanted directly into the tumor itself. These pellets, which are about the size of a grain of rice, attack the tumor while leaving nearby healthy tissue unharmed. The radioactive seeds remain inside the patient's body, delivering a low dose of radiation over a long period of time, thus the name low-dose-rate (LDR) brachytherapy.

Another method of brachytherapy utilizes temporary radioactive implants to attack the cancer. This type of therapy is called high-dose-rate (HDR) brachytherapy because the radioactive material used creates higher-intensity radiation than the cobalt 60 used in permanent implants. In HDR brachytherapy, several thin tubes are surgically placed through the patient's skin into the tumor. X-rays are taken to confirm the proper placement of the tubes in the tumor. Using computers, doctors determine the optimal dosage of radiation that will kill the tumor and produce the least harm to surrounding tissues. The patient is then taken to the treatment room, where the implanted tubes are attached to a machine called an afterloader. The afterloader, following the physician's computer instructions, automatically dispenses the radioactive pellets into the patient for the prescribed amount of time. When the procedure is completed, the radioactive pellets return to the afterloader, where they are safely stored.

There are many advantages in using HDR brachytherapy. The patient is exposed to the radiation for just

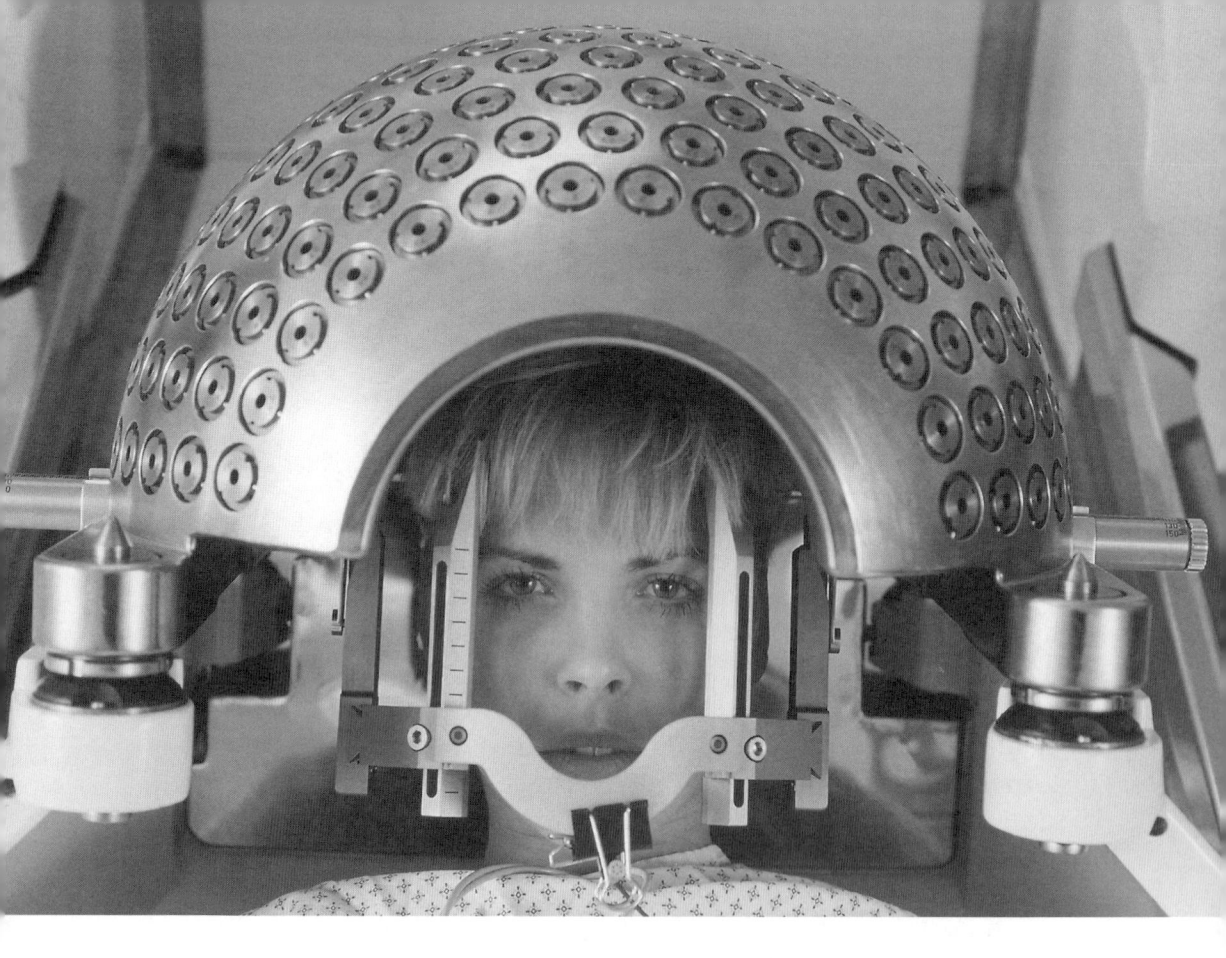

A child is outfitted with a Gamma Knife helmet covered with small holes that direct gamma radiation streams at cancerous tumors in his head.

minutes, rather than the long-term exposure associated with permanently implanted seeds. The amount of radiation the patient receives can be more precisely calculated than with implanted seeds, which may shift within the body and have a fixed amount of radiation that cannot be altered once implanted. In addition, since the procedure is automated using the afterloader, the risks of radiation exposure to doctors and technicians are minimized.

Advances in radiotherapy, both internal and external, have benefited many thousands of cancer patients who might otherwise have had to undergo traditional surgery with all its risks and side effects. Technological progress in medical imaging, meanwhile, has given the humble X-ray much clearer vision with which to probe the human body.

Chapter 5

Improving Medical Imaging

When William Randolph Hearst, publisher of the *New York Journal*, heard that Thomas Edison was experimenting with X-rays, he sent the inventor a telegram in February 1896:

WILL YOU AS AN ESPECIAL FAVOR TO THE JOURNAL UNDERTAKE TO MAKE A CATHODOGRAPH OF HUMAN BRAIN KINDLY TELEGRAPH ANSWER AT OUR EXPENSE.[36]

Always looking for a sensational piece of news for his publication, Hearst thought a "cathodograph," or X-ray, of a human brain would attract readers given the intense interest in the newly discovered rays. Edison agreed to Hearst's request, and for weeks reporters watched and waited as the inventor attempted to penetrate a human skull with X-rays. Despite all his efforts, Edison failed to produce an X-ray photograph of a brain. The X-rays of the day were just not strong enough to produce an acceptable result. In time, however, advancing technology in the fields of radiology and computers would reveal not only the human brain but also other internal structures never before visible with X-rays.

Scanning Pioneers

The idea of linking computers with X-ray machines to scan the interiors of objects was thought up by several researchers working independently and without knowledge of each other. In the 1950s and 1960s, astronomer Ronald Bracewell took telescopic images

Oldendorf's Forest

When William Oldendorf built his model scanning device, he used the example of a person in a forest to explain the theory behind its operation. Here is Oldendorf's explanation, as related by his widow in 1995, of his experiment that used nails, a model railroad car, and a gamma ray source. It is taken from Bettyann Holtzmann Kevles's book Naked to the Bone: Medical Imaging in the Twentieth Century:

An observer standing stationary in a forest might have a difficult time viewing a distant person because that person might be blocked by trees in between. But if the observer begins to move through the forest, while at the same time looking in the direction of the distant person, then the trees in the foreground would seem to move past, while the distant individual would seem to stay still. . . . The distant person represents the nails in the center of his model, and the trees [represent] the line of nails obscuring it. The observer's line of sight is like the gamma ray beam that is continuously pointed through the surrounding ring of nails at the interior nail. As the gamma source circles, the nails in front and behind the central nail momentarily absorb gamma rays, deleting them from the beam, creating the equivalent of the blurring motion of trees in the forest. The interior nail itself, located at the center of motion of the gamma ray source, absorbs gamma rays continuously.

William Oldendorf developed an X-ray scanning machine in the early 1960s.

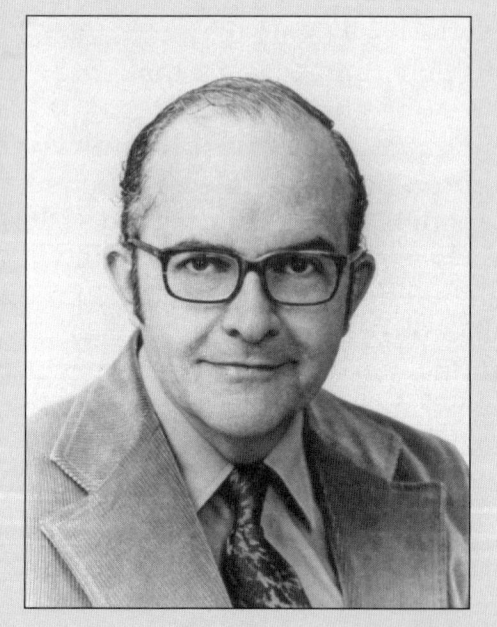

of the Sun and the Moon by obtaining one-dimensional data in strips and then using those data to create a two-dimensional map of the celestial objects. Bracewell's method of "slicing" and reconstructing information used radiotelescopes viewing outer space rather than X-ray machines viewing the inner body. But the mathematics involved in creating the images was eventually used in medical imaging.

Around the same time that Bracewell was photographing the Sun, William Oldendorf was practicing medicine at the Veterans Administration hospital in Los Angeles. As a neurologist interested in the workings of the human brain, Oldendorf was dissatisfied with the current methods of observing the brain's structure. Ordinary X-rays still could not produce a detailed image of the brain, and the process used, pneumoencephalography (making an X-ray by using air as a contrast medium), was painful for the patient. Even when Oldendorf directly x-rayed a brain that had been removed from a cadaver's skull, the resulting image was of poor quality. The reason for the difficulty in obtaining a satisfactory image of the brain lies in its physical makeup. It is almost uniformly dense, and as a result, X-rays have trouble differentiating between the various structures that lie within. The usual result was a poorly defined mass showing very little detail. Oldendorf knew there had to be a better way to obtain images from inside a structure such as the skull, and he finally found it in an unlikely object: an orange.

In 1958 Oldendorf happened to chat with an engineer who was trying to come up with a way to examine the inside of an orange in order to separate frostbitten fruit from good ones. Unfortunately, all oranges, good or bad, look about the same from the outside. The engineer thought of using an X-ray machine to scan the oranges. By rotating the X-ray beam around the orange, a scan could be created to measure the density within. The engineer never pursued this plan, but the idea fired Oldendorf's imagination. After all, an orange was similar to a human head, with a thick peel (the skull) protecting a delicate fruit (the brain) inside. Oldendorf went to his home workshop and came up with a model of a scanning X-ray machine using forty-two nails, a plastic block, a model train car and track, and a phonograph. Using gamma rays, Oldendorf's ingenious device was able to create a two-dimensional image of two target nails in the center of the plastic block while ignoring the other nails placed around the targets. Although the device was crude, it is the forerunner of today's medical scanners, incorporating virtually all the elements except a modern high-speed computer.

In 1961 Oldendorf published a paper on the findings of his experiments. He received a patent for the scanner in 1963, but he was unable to interest any companies in manufacturing it. One skeptical (and rather short-sighted) firm told him, "Even if it could be made to work as you suggest, we cannot imagine a significant market for such an expensive apparatus which would do nothing but make radiographic cross-sections of the head."[37] While Oldendorf went on to pursue other medical interests, a South African scientist was pondering the possibilities of mapping the body with X-rays.

Allan Cormack was one of the few nuclear physicists in South Africa in the 1950s. He worked a few days a week at Groote Schuur Hospital in Cape Town, where he supervised the use of radioactive isotopes in radiotherapy. While observing the methods used for planning radiotherapy treatments, Cormack decided that there should be a better way of measuring how the body absorbed radioactivity. He began experiments in South Africa and continued them after he moved to Boston to take a position at Tufts University. In 1963 Cormack built a prototype scanning device for about one hundred dollars. For a test subject, he constructed a model called a phantom to represent the human brain within the skull. Inside the model brain, he placed two aluminum disks representing tumors. His device created images that could detect within the test subject different densities, in this case the aluminum "tumors." Thus, Cormack was the first to actually create computerized tomographs—slices through an object. The word *computerized* might be exaggerating, for Cormack's computer was a simple desktop calculator.

Like Oldendorf, Cormack found little enthusiasm for his findings. In fact, the only inquiry came from scientists at the Swiss Avalanche Center, who wanted to know if his device could be used to measure the depth of snow on mountains. But the medical importance of Allan Cormack's work was vindicated when, in 1979, he won a Nobel Prize in physiology or medicine, an honor he shared with the man most often called the inventor of computerized axial tomography: Godfrey Newbold Hounsfield.

Hounsfield's Scanner

Godfrey Hounsfield was a genius, but he did poorly in the structured environment of school. Born in 1919 in Newark, England, young Hounsfield was more interested in doing experiments with homemade hang gliders and electrical devices than in attending to his schoolwork. Although he studied electrical engineering in college, he never received a PhD. But a college degree was less important to him than his love of experimenting and exploring new avenues of knowledge.

In 1951 Hounsfield went to work for EMI, Limited, a British corporation with interests in many fields but specializing in producing records. At EMI he performed research in the company's electronics division, where he was allowed to pursue whatever interested him. While he was working on computers that could scan a page of printed text, he wondered if such a computer could scan images as well as text. And what if those images were made by X-rays rather than ordinary light? His curious mind raced as he began to work on the problem in 1967.

As Allan Cormack had done a few years before, Hounsfield built prototype scanners using phantom targets and gamma rays as the radiation source. "The equipment was very much improvised," Hounsfield later recalled. "A lathe bed provided the lateral scanning movement of the gamma ray source, and sensitive detectors were placed on either side of the object to be viewed which was rotated one inch at the end of each sweep."[38] The results were encouraging but hardly prac-

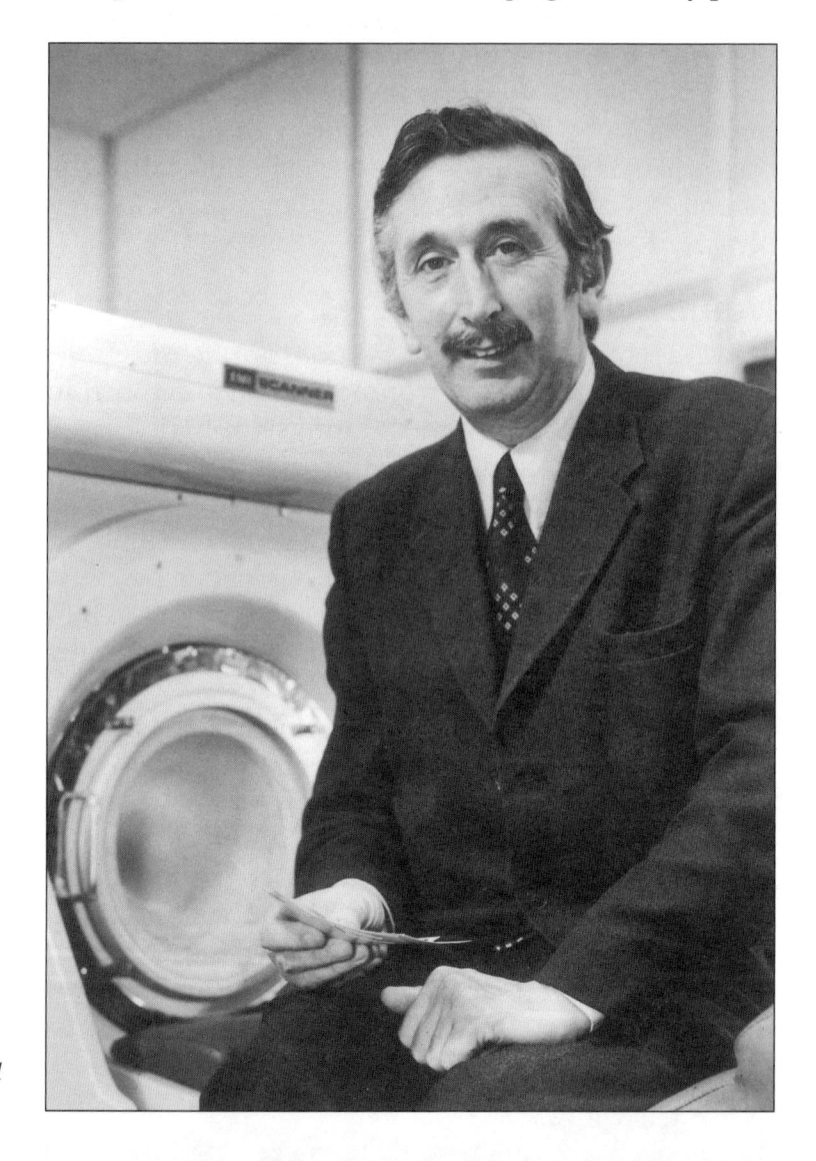

Godfrey Hounsfield poses with a CT scanner in 1979. Building on research conducted by South African physicist Allan Cormack, Hounsfield engineered the first CT scanner.

tical: It took nine days to perform a scan, and another two and a half hours for the computer to analyze the data and produce a picture. Switching to X-rays instead of gamma rays lowered the scan time to about nine hours. Further refinements were made until, on October 1, 1971, the first patient was scanned. After fifteen hours of scanning and the processing of twenty eight thousand readings, the resulting image clearly showed a tumor in the patient's brain. The next year EMI began commercial production of the computed axial tomography scanner. At first designed to scan only the brain, in a few years scanners were able to scan any part of the body. At the Nobel Prize ceremony in 1979, Hounsfield met Allan Cormack for the first time as they shared the award in physiology or medicine.

How Scanners Work

Computed axial tomography (abbreviated CAT scan, although now usually referred to as a CT—computed tomography—scan) brings the scanning principle developed by Jean Kieffer in the 1920s into the computer age. The main parts of a CT scanner are the X-ray tube and the X-ray detectors. The tube produces the X-rays that pass through the patient's body; where the X-rays strike the detectors, small flashes of light are converted into electrical pulses. These components are mounted opposite each other inside a large, ring-shaped assembly called a gantry, which looks like a huge doughnut sitting on its side.

The patient receiving the scan lies down on a movable table, which slowly slides into the "hole" of the doughnut. Then the X-ray tube and detectors begin to rotate around the patient, scanning a slice of the body only a fraction of an inch thick. During each rotation, data from the electrical pulses generated by X-rays striking the detectors is stored in a computer. After a complete rotation, the table moves slightly farther into the hole and another slice is scanned. The process continues until the body portion of interest to the

Computed Tomography (CT) Scanner

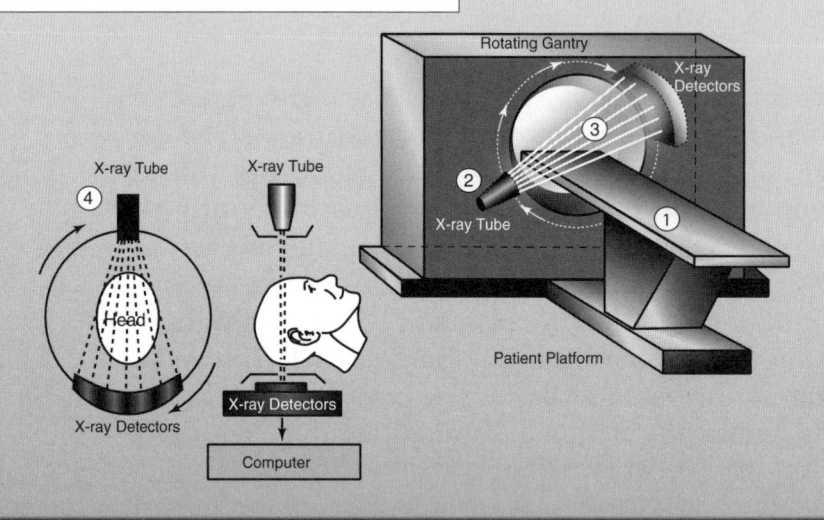

A CT scanning machine uses X-rays and computers to form a three-dimensional model of a patient's bones, organs, and other interior body parts.

1. The patient lies on a platform which slowly moves through a hole in the center of the scanning machine.

2. Around the hole is a rotating frame called a gantry, with an X-ray tube mounted on one side and an arc-shaped array of X-ray detectors mounted directly opposite.

3. The X-ray tube emits a fan-shaped beam of X-rays as the gantry spins around the patient. About one thousand images are created with each rotation. Each time the gantry makes a 360° rotation, one slice is created.

4. The gantry rotates around the patient until all the data is gathered. Computers process all of the information and create a three-dimensional image of the scanned body part.

physicians (the brain, for example) is completely scanned— sometimes as many as fifteen hundred slices. Then the computer reconstructs the information it received from the scans to create images of the slices of the body. These images present doctors with a clear view of the inside of the body, detailed enough to detect tumors and other defects.

In a scan of the brain, the skull, being most opaque to X-rays, appears white. The structure of the brain itself is displayed as various shades of gray, revealing its various densities. Black areas on a scan indicate the cerebrospinal fluid, a clear liquid that fills the spinal cord and the cavities in the brain. As with standard radiography, a contrast medium is sometimes injected into the patient through an intravenous tube in order to make a more detailed study of the brain. Scanners are also used for examining the lungs, liver, kidneys, and other internal organs that do not show up clearly on ordinary X-rays. The vascular system, the veins and arteries that transport blood throughout the body, can also be examined by CT using a contrast medium.

As the technology of CT scanners advanced, new machines and methods of scanning were developed. These advances resulted in new "generations" of CT scanners. The original, or first-generation, scanners utilized one X-ray source and one detector that rotated in unison to produce images. Further developments resulted in second-generation machines that added more X-ray detectors, increasing the speed of the scans. Third-generation scanners utilized even more detectors, and by the fourth generation, X-ray detectors encircled the patient in a 360-degree ring. The patient rests at the center of the ring, and the X-ray source spins around the patient, revolving just inside the X-ray detector ring.

The Pros and Cons of CT

There are several advantages of computed tomography over ordinary X-rays. CT scans can differentiate soft body structures that a regular X-ray cannot. In fact, CTs can detect a difference in what is called the attenuation rate—the amount of x-radiation that is absorbed, or attenuated, by various body structures—ten times better than with ordinary X-rays. This is critical for examining the soft tissues of the body. Body structures that may obstruct the area or organ under examination do not affect the contrast of the CT scan and thus do not obscure the image as would occur in an ordinary X-ray. In addition, increased resolution and less visual "noise," or interference that decreases the quality of an image, make CT scans the method of choice for numerous diagnostic applications.

Nonetheless, there are some disadvantages to using CT scanners. The radiation dose received by the patient

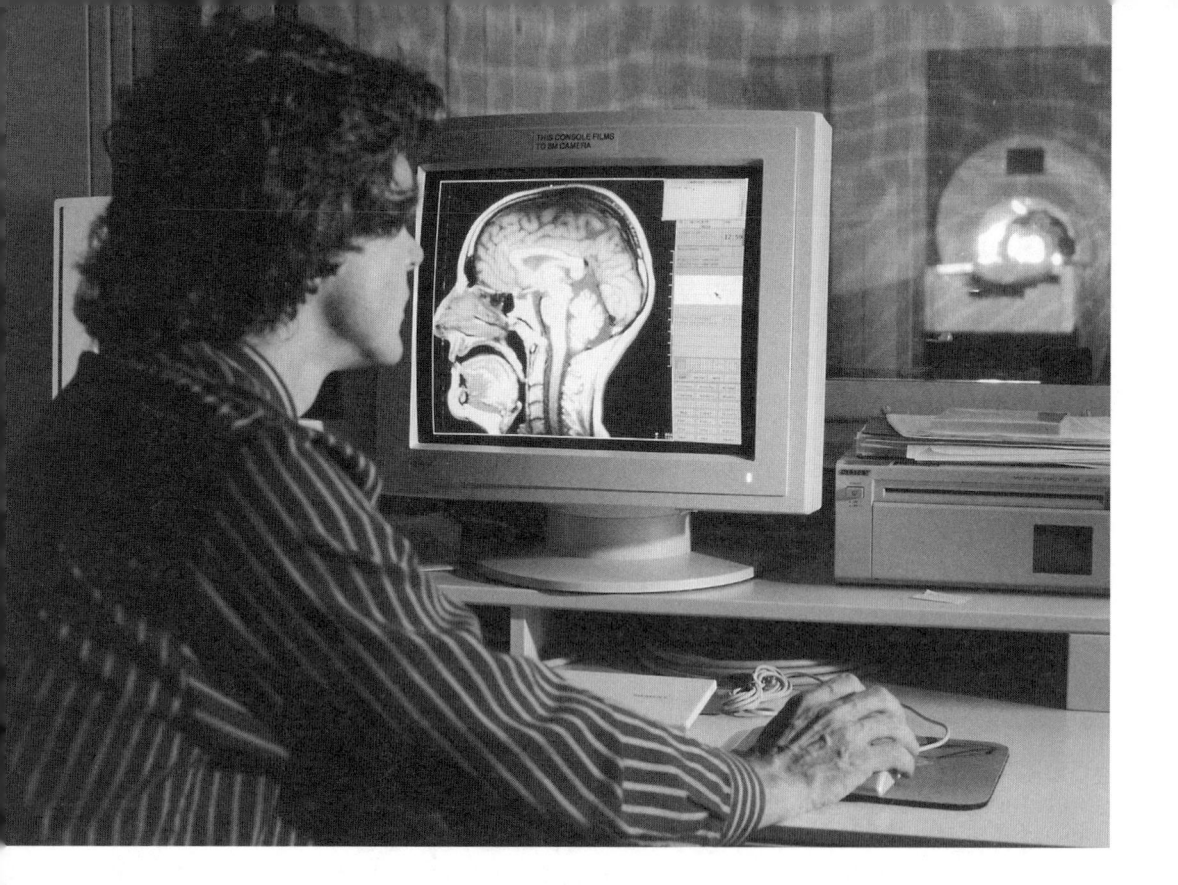

A medical assistant examines a cross-section of a patient's head as the patient moves through a CT scanner in the adjoining room.

is higher than with standard X-rays. But this risk must be weighed against the amount of information gained when diagnosing life-threatening illnesses. CT scans are generally more expensive than regular X-rays due to the cost of scanning equipment and related computer software (scanners can cost more than $1 million). Sometimes, CT scans will create "artifacts," or false information, that may distort the final image.

Despite these disadvantages, the CT scan has become a standard method of diagnosis. Another method of seeing inside the body is similar to computed tomography, but it differs in one important point: it involves no X-rays at all.

Diagnosis by Magnetism

In the 1940s physicists discovered that by subjecting spinning atoms to a strong magnetic field their nuclei would wobble around their magnetic axis, the same way a spinning top will wobble if you gently nudge it with your finger. This phenomenon provided the

Improving Medical Imaging

basis for an advanced kind of medical imaging called magnetic resonance imaging (MRI).

An MRI scanner is a large machine similar in appearance and layout to a CT scanner. The MRI "doughnut" is deeper than that of a CT scanner, allowing the entire body to enter the machine. Inside the doughnut are coils of wire that form an extremely powerful electromagnet. During an MRI exam, the patient lies down on a movable table and is drawn into the scanner. The electromagnet generates a strong magnetic field that causes the nuclei of hydrogen atoms in the patient's

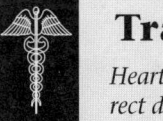

Tracking Heart Disease

Heart disease is the number-one killer in America. While surgery can often correct defects in the heart and its associated arteries, it is a costly and risky procedure. With magnetic resonance imaging (MRI), however, doctors can examine the heart and determine if surgery is necessary. Here, from the RadiologyInfo.org Web site, is an overview of cardiac MRI.

Magnetic resonance imaging is becoming very important in the initial diagnosis and subsequent management of coronary heart disease. MRI can help physicians to look closely at the structures and function of the heart and major vessels quickly and thoroughly, without the risks associated with traditional, more invasive procedures.

After a heart attack . . . an MRI examination can help the cardiologist understand how well the heart is pumping, whether the flow of blood is blocked in any chamber or major vessel, whether the heart muscles are damaged, or whether the lining of the heart is swelling. This is critical knowledge needed to administer prompt and effective treatment. MRI can also detect the buildup of plaque and blockages in the blood vessels, making it an invaluable tool for detecting and evaluating coronary artery disease.

An MRI scan gives doctors a complete image of a patient's heart and circulatory system.

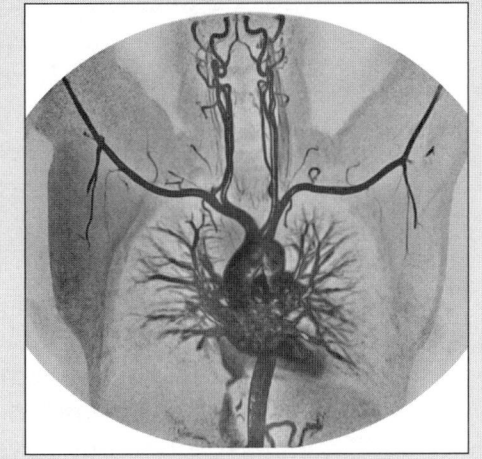

body to wobble. Radio frequency (RF) waves are then beamed through the patient's body, much like X-rays are beamed in a CT scan. When the RF waves are turned off, the nuclei emit their own weak RF energy, which is recorded as data in a computer. The computer then assembles the data into pictures, which display slices of the interior of the patient's body.

The magnetic resonance imaging scanner was developed by Raymond Damadian, a physician who received his medical degree in 1960. After experimenting with magnetic resonance on bacteria, he thought the same technique might be used to detect cancer in humans. He reasoned that if the nuclei of cancer cells and healthy cells emit distinctive RF patterns, the difference would indicate the presence of a tumor. Experiments with rats proved Damadian correct, and he published his findings in 1971. He then went about developing a scanner that could scan a living body with magnetic and radio waves. On July 3, 1977, the first MRI scan of a human (one of Damadian's colleagues) was made.

The Pros and Cons of MRI

One of the biggest advantages of magnetic resonance imaging is that, unlike standard X-rays or CT scans, it uses no radiation. The magnetic field and RF waves employed by MRI have not been shown to have any harmful effects on living tissue. Another advantage is that MRI scans can be made at unlimited angles through the body, whereas CT scans can only scan the body axially (like slices in a loaf of bread). Images of soft tissues in the body are more detailed in an MRI.

There are, however, some drawbacks to MRI. The electromagnets used in an MRI scanner can generate a magnetic field some thirty thousand times stronger than Earth's own magnetic field. People who have any metal in their bodies (such as surgical clips or artificial joints) cannot undergo an MRI exam. Some people suffer from claustrophobia, the fear of enclosed spaces, and may not be able to tolerate being in the MRI scanner for the period necessary for the scan to take place. In these cases, a mild sedative may be administered to relax the patient and calm his or her anxiety.

Imaging the Body

X-rays, computed tomography, and magnetic resonance imaging have all had a profound effect on the way diseases are diagnosed and on the way people think about medical diagnosis. In the United States, millions of scans are performed each year. Twenty million X-rays and CT and MRI scans are used annually just to diagnose cancer. Pictures of the body's interior structure no longer produce awe and wonder in the minds of the public, as they did at the beginning of the twentieth century. Patients and doctors alike consider scans to be routine tools at the physician's disposal. For many patients, diagnostic imaging has taken the place of exploratory surgery, saving them from having dangerous and invasive procedures. Doctors routinely use CT and MRI scans to guide them during surgical procedures.

Medical imaging has not been without its adversaries, however. As CT scanners began to filter into the medical community, their enormous cost caused concern that health care would become too expensive. For most hospitals, being able to offer the latest technology to patients meant better health care, but it also meant having to attract more patients in order to generate more income. In the 1970s the federal government became concerned that too many hospitals were buying expensive scanners, raising costs while merely duplicating the services of other nearby hospitals. In 1976 Secretary of Health, Education, and Welfare Joseph Califano reportedly commented that "every hospital no more needed a CT scanner than every garage needed a Cadillac."[39] Certificate-of-need (CON) laws were passed requiring hospitals to obtain state approval for big-budget purchases. This often led to frustration and delays in purchasing needed equipment. Even today,

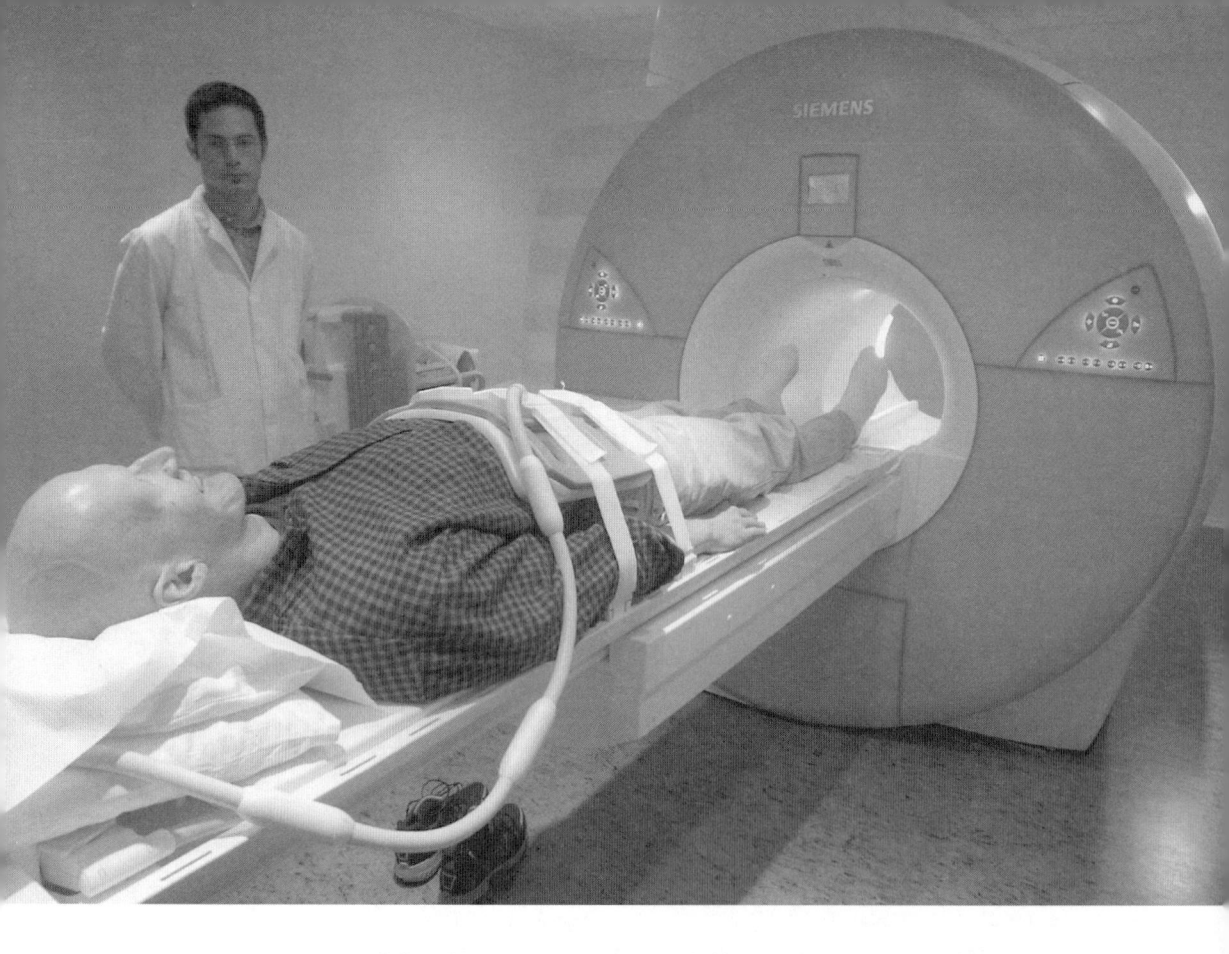

A cancer patient is introduced into an MRI scanning tube. MRI scans and other diagnostic imaging technologies help doctors diagnose diseases without invasive surgery.

CON laws can make it difficult for medical facilities to upgrade their technology. Journalist Jean P. Fisher examined North Carolina's CON laws and found that "when hospitals and physician practices see a need for, say, more scanners for magnetic resonance imaging, or MRIs, they can't even apply for one until the state's number crunchers see the need, too."[40] As a result of these restrictions, the introduction of MRI scanners by U.S. medical facilities proceeded more slowly than did the earlier CT scanners.

Some critics say that physicians may be tempted to order too many or unnecessary scans as a way to pay back the large initial cost of the technology. Others maintain that increased reliance on high-tech machinery may imperil the doctor-patient relationship that is so important to good health care. Brian Lentle, a Canadian radiologist, no doubt echoes the sentiments of most doctors as he refutes this latter claim: "Our compassionate behaviour as physicians is unlikely to be hindered by having up-to-date tools and may indeed be helped by them."[41]

Medical imaging in today's hospital is a technological marvel unlike anything Wilhelm Röntgen could have imagined. In less than a hundred years, X-rays went from a novelty (and a dangerous one at that) to a vital part of health care. The twenty-first century is sure to produce even more amazing technological advances. Indeed, the seeds of future technology are being sown today by forward-thinking researchers, manufacturers, and physicians.

Chapter 6

Images of the Future

X-rays have long played a part in the world of science fiction. In 1897, just two years after Wilhelm Röntgen made his discovery, a pioneering French filmmaker produced a short, fanciful movie in which a skeleton leaves a body when x-rayed by a doctor. A British film that same year also incorporated the new X-rays: As two lovers sat on a park bench, an X-ray beam revealed their bones. By the 1930s, Superman was a familiar figure in the comics, fighting for justice with the help of his X-ray vision. A long list of television shows and movies have kept the Man of Steel's extraordinary powers entertaining audiences worldwide. Through comics, novels, and films, science fiction fans have become familiar with deadly "ray guns" and other fictional uses of radiation.

But beyond the world of science fiction, real scientists are developing fantastic new uses for X-rays. In the ever-changing field of medical technology, X-ray machines and the science of radiology will continue to evolve in ways that would surprise even the most creative science fiction writers.

Full-Body Scanning

In 1896 people were fascinated (and sometimes frightened) at seeing the bones in their hands as they visited Thomas Edison's fluoroscope display at the New

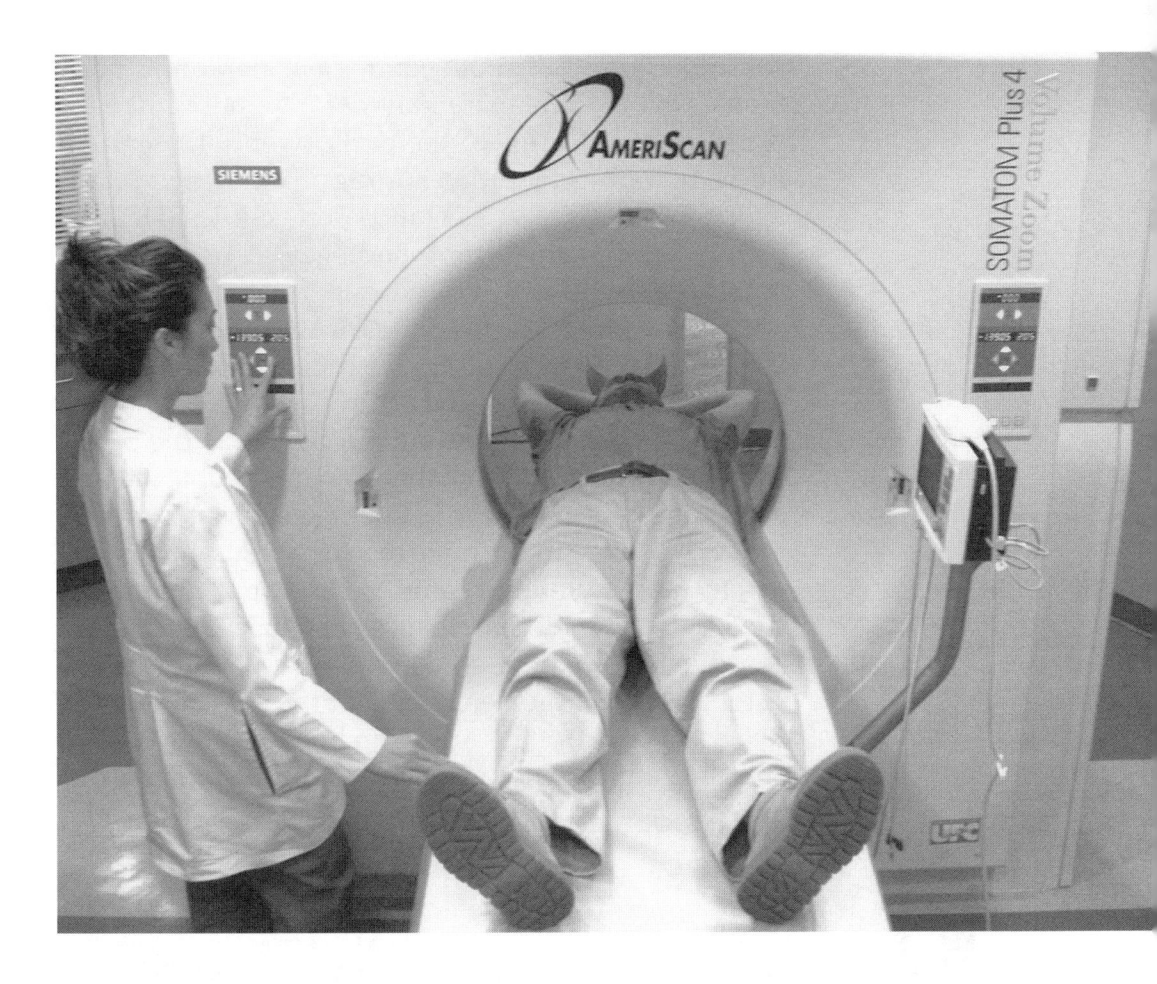

York electrical exhibition. For most of its existence, radiology has been used to examine specific parts of the body in an effort to diagnose a particular disease, locate foreign objects in the body, or examine bone fractures. In the mid-1990s, however, examining the entire body by X-ray appeared to be the next step in the evolution of X-rays. Full-body scans utilize computed tomography to x-ray a large portion of the body, usually from neck to hips. Proponents of this procedure say it can discover certain diseases when they are most curable. "We can save lives," comments Kenneth Cooper, a doctor with the Cooper Clinic, a full-body scan facility near Dallas, Texas. "With the full-body CT scan, we can pick up heart disease and cancer at their

A patient undergoes a full-body CT scan at a shopping mall. Proponents of full-body scans contend that the technology is able to detect cancers at their earliest stages.

earliest stages."[42] Through aggressive marketing, body scans soon became extremely popular, not unlike the X-ray photo studios of the early twentieth century. Body-scanning facilities sprang up in office parks, shopping malls, and as stand-alone clinics. Healthy people without any symptoms began requesting body scans, hoping to detect diseases before warning signs appeared. Some 32 million scans were performed in 2002. It seemed as if full-body scans would emerge as the diagnostic wave of the future.

Critics soon began voicing opposition to the procedure. It was not necessary, they said, for people without any symptoms of disease to undergo such an extensive —and expensive (often more than one thousand dollars) —screening. Full-body scans can find small anomalies such as cysts and scars, that may be harmless and yet could lead to patient anxiety or, worse, unnecessary surgery. "In a large percentage of the cases," says Dr. Robert J. Stanley of the American Roentgen Ray Society, "these things are not worthy of being evaluated fur-

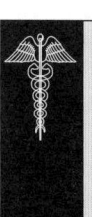

The Ethics of Medical Imaging

As medical imaging advances into uncharted territory, questions about the ethical use of this technology are sure to arise. In a 1995 article in the journal World Health, *Dr. Sneh Bhargava discusses the ethics of advanced medical technology.*

There is no doubt that the radiological and imaging sciences have made unprecedented progress from simple X-ray films to the era of anatomical scans.... Such scans... have brought such precision and confidence to medical diagnosis as never before and are actively involved in every field of medicine from the unborn fetus to the brain dead. So much for the positive side.

On the negative side, they have changed medicine from being an art with a human face to that of a complex science with a dollar value. Their rising costs have increased the gap between the haves and the have-nots in terms of the availability of quality health care. The most vulnerable, the poor and those who are most in need of health care are getting less and less. The new technologies have usurped limited resources, away from preventive health care and primary health care—in part because of the powerful lobbies that industry has created among the medical administrators.

ther."[43] In some cases the opposite may occur: A patient given a clean bill of health after a body scan might neglect other standard tests designed to detect specific diseases. Another concern is the increased amount of radiation received by a patient during a full-body scan. A 2004 study by the journal *Radiology* found that a full-body radiation dose "is comparable to the doses received by some of the atomic bomb survivors from Hiroshima and Nagasaki, where there is clear evidence of increased cancer risk."[44] Proponents of full-body scans argue that the test is a valuable diagnostic tool, and they have testimonials from patients whose cancer was diagnosed early and treated successfully.

Advocates of the full-body scan say that the radiation hazard has not been proven, whereas opponents argue that neither has the effectiveness of the scans. While the full-body scan debate continues, a perhaps more promising technology has X-rays looking at some of the human body's smallest elements.

Molecular Imaging

Traditional X-rays, CT scans, and MRI scans reveal to physicians the structures of the human body and whether there are any signs of disease present in those structures. While the most sophisticated scanners can detect extremely small abnormalities, there is a lot going on in the body on an even smaller scale. What if doctors could look inside a living cell and observe its molecules as they go about their jobs of creating the biological processes of that cell that, in turn, sustain the life of the body? Molecular imaging lets physicians do just that. Researchers predict a promising future for molecular imaging in the understanding of cells, how they work, and how they become diseased.

Molecular imaging uses a technology called positron emission tomography (PET). In the 1950s scientists in the United States were exploring the possibilities of scanning patients using positrons, which are identical to electrons but carry a positive rather than a negative electrical charge. This type of scanning was called emission tomography because it tracked the emissions of a radioactive source inside the body. Progress on emission scanning was slow until the early 1970s, when scientists discovered that the mathematical calculations used for creating images in Godfrey Hounsfield's CT scanners (which was "transmission" tomography because it passed, or transmitted, rays through the body) were useful for emission scanning as well. Once this realization was made, development of positron scanning machines could move forward.

Looking somewhat like a CT machine, the PET scanner has a ring of gamma-ray sensors in its "doughnut" rather than a moving X-ray source and detectors. A solution of glucose (sugar) mixed with a small amount of a radioactive substance is injected into the patient undergoing the scan. As the solution enters the part of the body being examined (the brain, for example), it gives off positrons. When the positrons enter the brain, they collide with the electrons that are already there; as a result, gamma rays are given off and detected by the scanner's sensors. A computer then assembles the information from the scanner into images.

PET scans are valuable because they can detect chemical changes in cells before structural changes are apparent, leading to earlier diagnosis and better management of cancer and heart disease. Because PET scans can show whether cells are growing or dying, it can reveal if chemotherapy is killing cancer cells in a tumor or if new cells are being created in a diseased heart. Therapy then can be adjusted to maximize its effect on the disease. A new innovation in medical imaging is the PET/CT scanner, a machine that combines images from both technologies to create clearer pictures of the size, shape, and growth activity of cancerous tumors, helping doctors combat the disease more effectively. In the future, PET scans will help fight major diseases in one of the fastest growing segments of the population: the elderly.

An Elder Nation

The baby boom is generally defined as the population explosion that occurred between 1946 and 1964. During that period nearly 76 million babies were born. This was a remarkable increase compared to a similar period of their parents' generation, when some 50 million babies were born between 1915 and 1933. For the last several decades, the elderly population in the United States has been growing faster than the population as a whole, and by the year 2030 one in five people will be over the age of sixty-five (compared to one in eight in 1994). As the baby boomers age, diseases of the elderly will become more and more of a strain on the American health care system. It is estimated that 80 percent of illnesses occur during the last 20 percent of a person's life.

One of the most devastating afflictions of the elderly is Alzheimer's disease, a progressive and irreversible disease caused by the degeneration of brain cells. In 2004 some 4 million people were afflicted with Alzheimer's, a number that will increase as the population ages. "Deterioration in people's brains usually begins five or ten years before they exhibit symptoms,"[45] says biomedical researcher Nadeem Ishaque. But new methods

These PET scans show dramatically reduced activity and blood flow in the brain of an Alzheimer's patient (right) compared to the brain of a healthy person (left).

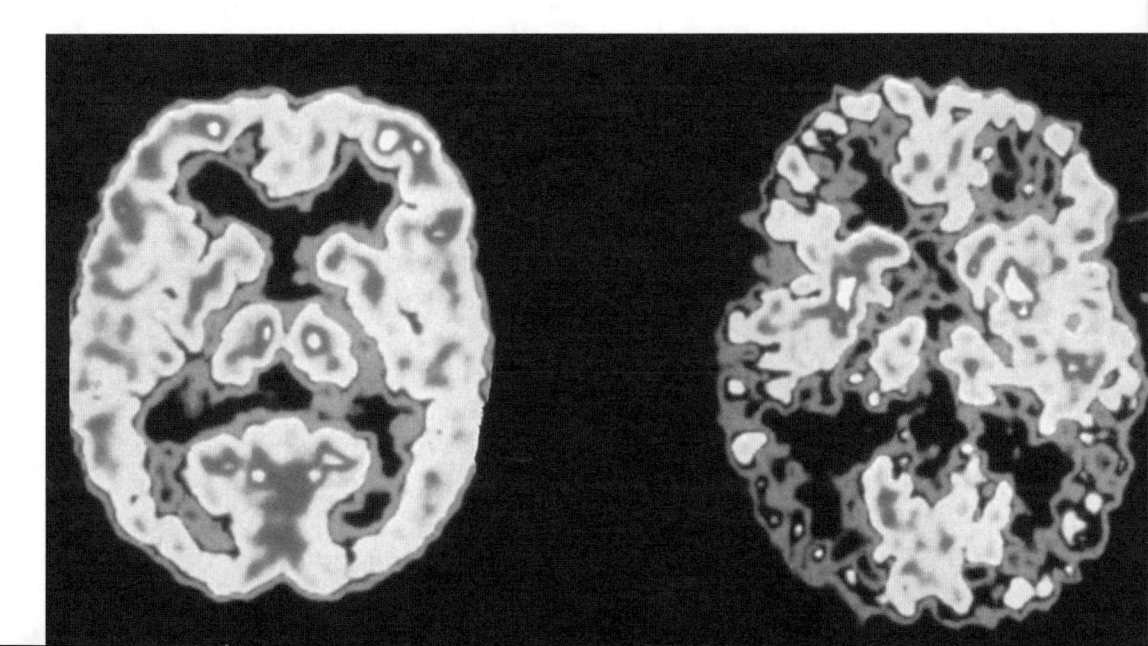

of brain imaging may help scientists discover the cause of the disease, choose the proper treatment, and ultimately develop a cure. Biomarkers are biological indicators of a process or condition in a living organism. For example, gray hair can be called a biomarker for aging. Molecular biomarkers can indicate the onset of a disease long before symptoms appear. By imaging the molecular biomarkers for Alzheimer's disease with PET scans, doctors can prescribe treatment that may slow the progression of the illness. "The imaging of biomarkers," notes Dr. Michael Phelps of the University of California, Los Angeles, "will provide a diagnosis based on how cells have been reprogrammed into disease. This helps establish new ways for how molecular therapeutics are developed, drugs are selected for patients, and therapeutic responses are assessed."[46] Using further PET scans to follow the progress of Alzheimer's once it has been diagnosed can track the effectiveness of drugs administered.

The technology is still developing and has led to debates on the PET scan's effectiveness in diagnosing Alzheimer's disease. Some say that there is no definitive test for the disease, but others report results with better than 90-percent accuracy in diagnosing Alzheimer's. Further research in imaging will ultimately determine the true value of PET scanning in the fight against Alzheimer's disease.

X-rays Without Film

In the mid-1990s a revolution in photography was beginning to take place. Digital cameras, which could take pictures without using traditional film, began appearing in camera stores. These cameras use charge-coupled devices (CCDs) to convert light into digital images that are recorded on a memory card and can be viewed on a computer screen or printed. With its convenience, versatility, and economy (no more paying for film and developing), digital photography soon surpassed film photography in popularity. A similar rev-

Images of the Future

olution is taking place in medical imaging, and doctors viewing large X-ray films on light boxes in darkened rooms may become a thing of the past.

Picture archive and communication systems (PACS) make storing, retrieving, and sharing X-rays much more timely and convenient for physicians. Using PACS, images generated by X-ray, MRI, CT, and PET scanners are digitized and stored in a hospital's main computer system. Once in the system, images are immediately available and may be accessed via computer terminal by any doctor in the hospital. In an emergency, such fast access to medical images can mean the difference between life and death. Of course, this archive system is a valuable technology even in routine cases. For example, an oncologist, or cancer specialist, can conduct consultations with a referring physician without having to wait for X-ray films to be delivered to his or

A doctor examines digital X-rays on a computer screen. Computerized X-rays make it much easier for physicians to share images with one another.

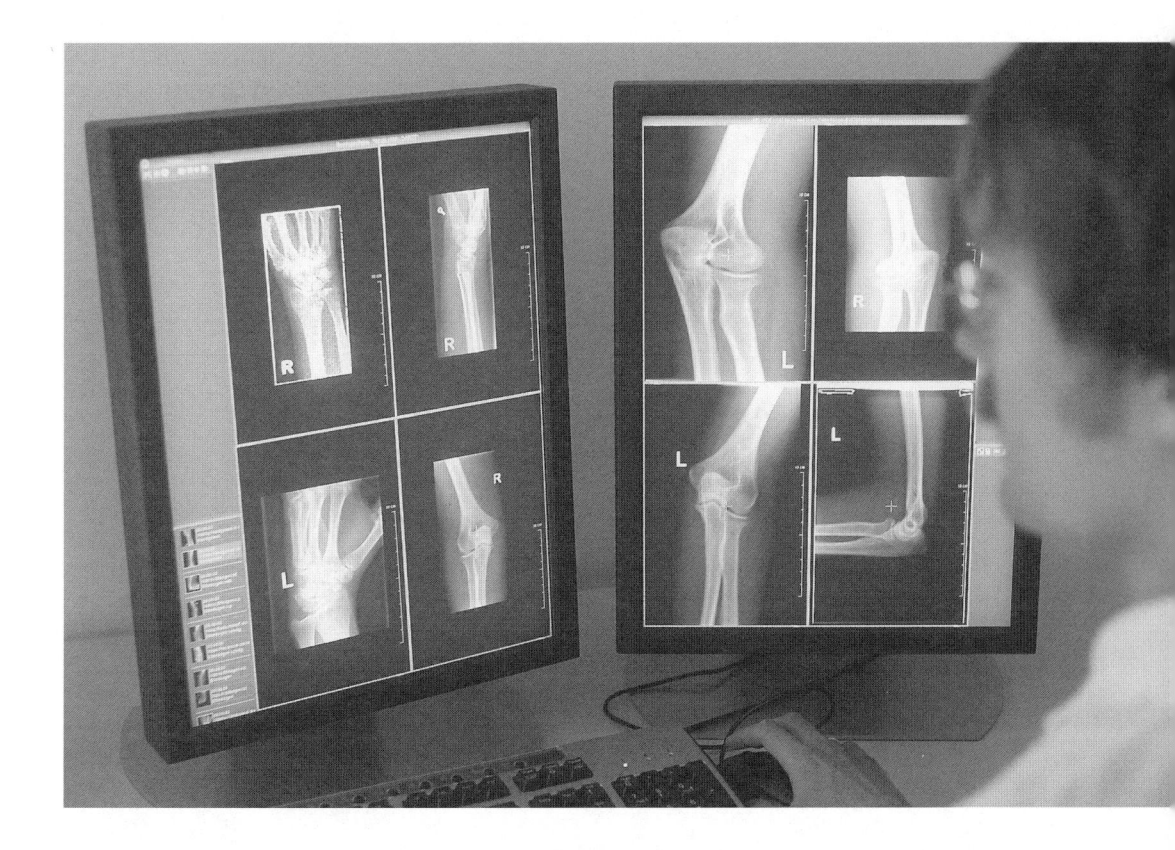

her office. And the PAC system is not limited to the departments within a hospital. Any number of doctors across the United States or around the world can conduct conferences via telephone while viewing the medical images on their own computers. Other advantages include the fact that digital images cannot be lost or misplaced and that images can be adjusted on individual computer screens for optimum clarity.

As with any such change in technology, problems can occur. For example, physicians and X-ray technicians will need to be trained to use the PAC system. Installing such a complicated system involves weighing many factors: cost, workflow efficiency, improvement of patient outcomes, and the diagnostic accuracy of viewing images on a computer screen. In addition, technical support and maintenance become critical elements in systems where a computer crash can prevent life-saving information from reaching a doctor. But the true advantage of the PACS lies in more than just increased accessibility. According to Paul Chang, director of radiology informatics at the University of Pittsburgh, "Everyone thinks the goal of PACS is to get images everywhere, but that's only half the puzzle.... The real goal is not just to disseminate information everywhere but to eliminate isolation and create an environment of collaboration by combining infrastructure with collaborative tools."[47]

Remote Medicine

The Internet has affected nearly all aspects of modern life. But as digital technology advances, the Internet can seem like a horse and buggy in a Ferrari world when it comes to downloading massive files of data and pictures. The future of the online transfer of medical images may lie in the realm of Internet2. Created by a nonprofit consortium of some three hundred universities and technology companies, Internet2 could be the future of broadband Internet applications. Compared to broadband connections that can handle

> ### X-rays in an Instant
>
> *In large hospitals, hundreds of X-rays may be taken every day. Such a huge workload may be eased by technological advances, such as the futuristic scene described in the online article "Smart Technology: Aiding Diagnosis and Productivity" from the Medical Imaging.org Web site:*
>
> Picture a digital imaging detector built into a stretcher in an ambulance. In the few critical moments before reaching the hospital, emergency personnel take X-rays of the patient. The images, beamed wirelessly to the hospital, enable the emergency room staff to begin treatment immediately upon arrival. Using organic electronics, scientists are expanding flexibility in the capture of X-rays. Such technology may be embedded in a hospital bed, a wheelchair, or even a hospital gown, enabling X-rays to be taken with minimal inconvenience to the patient. In addition, such devices free up hospital resources by eliminating the need to transport patients.

around 500 Kbps (500,000 bits of information per second), Internet2 can download information at a blazing 10 Gbps (10 billion bits per second) over thirteen thousand miles of fiberoptic cable. By 2004 only about 10 to 15 percent of Internet2 was being used—obviously, there is much room for growth.

Speed, reliability, and what is called "quality of service" will make the future Internet ideal for sharing medical images. Wireless technology, connecting computers to the Internet without physical cables, will also help get health information where it is needed most. The screens of early twenty-first-century wireless devices, such as laptop computers and personal digital assistants (PDAs), lack sufficient resolution to make them very useful for medical imaging. But in the future, technology will overcome such limitations. "There will be full diagnostic resolution laptops," comments Aaron Waitz of Kodak Health Imaging, "but in 2020, your computer will be the size of your PDA and you are either going to have a flexible monitor that you unroll and lay down on a table for viewing, or you'll wear special eyeglasses that will project the image directly onto your retina."[48] Recent research has shown that PDAs hold promise for future radiologists. "Our first study," says

This detailed full-body image was taken by an experimental MRI scanner that could become a common diagnostic tool in the very near future.

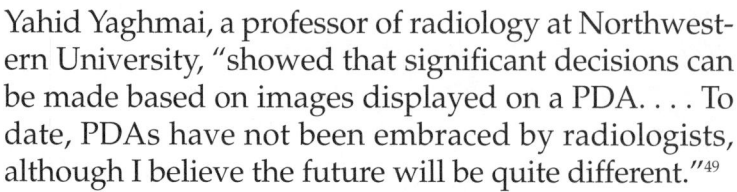

Yahid Yaghmai, a professor of radiology at Northwestern University, "showed that significant decisions can be made based on images displayed on a PDA.... To date, PDAs have not been embraced by radiologists, although I believe the future will be quite different."[49]

Telemedicine is the term for using high-speed computer networks to send medical information to remote areas that do not have the latest in diagnostic equipment or expertise. Through such technologies as videoconferencing and real-time data transmission, patients can get help they might never have gotten before. For example, a patient on the Pacific island of Guam underwent delicate heart surgery supervised by a surgeon thirty-five hundred miles away in Honolulu, Hawaii.

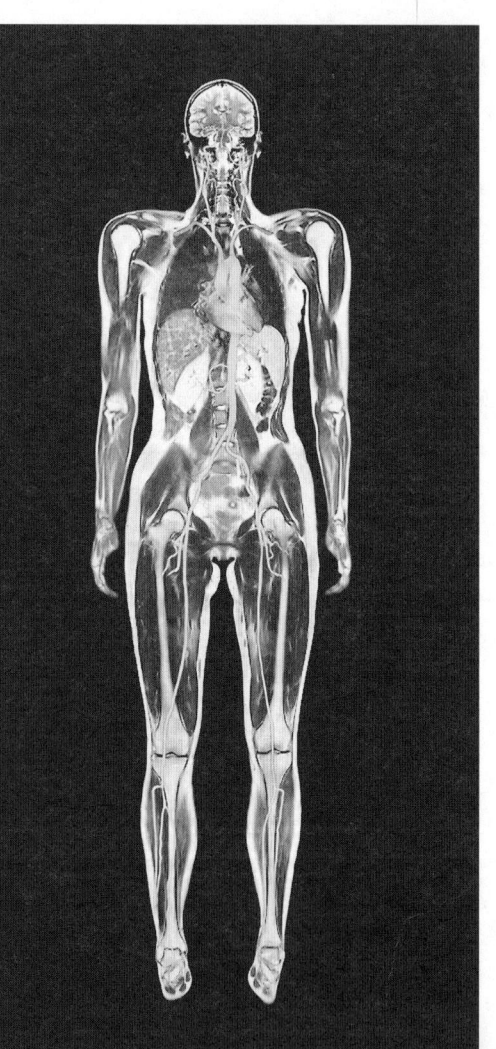

Teleradiology is the specialty of sending medical images through a computer network for diagnosis and consultation. Many large hospitals offer teleradiology services twenty-four hours a day for doctors offices or clinics that take X-rays but do not have a radiologist on staff to interpret the images. This service is especially important in emergency cases that occur at night, a time when studies show there are increasing requests for X-ray interpretation. Doctors who provide such after-hours X-ray readings are sometimes called nighthawks, and their numbers are increasing. Using a nighthawk to interpret X-rays is valuable to a hospital not only monetarily but also in saving its own radiologists from the added burden of working extra night shifts. Often nighthawks will work in locales where, when it is nighttime in the United States, it is day where the radiologist is on call. For example, an X-ray transmitted at midnight from California would be displayed on a nighthawk's computer in Sydney, Australia, at 4:00 in the afternoon. As the number of medical images generated by hospitals grows in the future, the use of teleradiology will become an increasingly valuable service for physicians.

Beyond Tomorrow

As digital technology advances in the twenty-first century, medical imaging will grow as well. The manufacturing of diagnostic medical imaging equipment was a $13.4 billion industry in 2000, and it is expected to have grown some 7 percent annually by 2006. The number of freestanding imaging centers, such as open MRI facilities, continues to expand as more and more procedures are performed outside the confines of a traditional hospital. Doctors are presented with clearer and more detailed images with which to diagnose their patients. Patients, in turn, can use the Internet to become more knowledgeable about their illnesses and treatment options. Technological advances often seem to come straight out of science fiction, such as smart technology that will track a doctor's eye movements as he or she looks at an X-ray. This technology determines which portions of an X-ray attract a doctor's attention. Then it asks if the physician would like to study those areas further.

Imaging equipment has become faster, more accurate, less expensive, and more patient friendly. The main result of these factors is an increase in the early detection, and therefore improved treatment, of such life-threatening illnesses as cancer and heart disease. Will medical science one day be able to vanquish these diseases, and the numerous other serious illnesses that plague humankind? If so, it will be with the help of the many descendants of Wilhelm Conrad Röntgen's marvelous discovery, X-rays.

Notes

Chapter 1: Diagnosing Disease

1. Quoted in Roy Porter, ed., *The Cambridge Illustrated History of Medicine*. Cambridge, UK: Cambridge University Press, 1996, p. 54.
2. Quoted in Porter, *The Cambridge Illustrated History of Medicine*, p. 159.
3. Quoted in Center for the Study of Technology and Society, "Today in Technology History: February 22." www.tecsoc.org/pubs/history/2002/feb22.htm.
4. Stanley Joel Reiser, *Medicine and the Reign of Technology*. Cambridge, UK: Cambridge University Press, 1978, pp. 2–3.
5. Quoted in Reiser, *Medicine and the Reign of Technology*, p. 23.
6. Quoted in Reiser, *Medicine and the Reign of Technology*, p. 25.
7. Reiser, *Medicine and the Reign of Technology*, p. 2.
8. Quoted in Reiser, *Medicine and the Reign of Technology*, p. 47.

Chapter 2: Wilhelm Röntgen's "New Rays"

9. Quoted in Vivian Grey, *Roentgen's Revolution: The Discovery of the X Ray*. Boston: Little, Brown, 1973, p. 23.
10. Quoted in Grey, *Roentgen's Revolution*, p. 35.
11. Quoted in Grey, *Roentgen's Revolution*, p. 69.
12. Quoted in W. Robert Nitske, "*The Life of Wilhelm Conrad Röntgen, Discoverer of the X Ray*. Tucson: University of Arizona Press, 1971, p. 4.

13. Quoted in Otto Glasser, *William Conrad Röntgen and the Early History of the Röntgen Rays*. Springfield, IL: Charles C. Thomas, 1934, p. 6.
14. Quoted in Glasser, *William Conrad Röntgen and the Early History of the Röntgen Rays*, p. 48.
15. Quoted in Nitske, *The Life of Wilhelm Conrad Röntgen, Discoverer of the X Ray*, p. 5.
16. Quoted in Nitske, *The Life of Wilhelm Conrad Röntgen, Discoverer of the X Ray*, p. 6.
17. Quoted in Nitske, *The Life of Wilhelm Conrad Röntgen, Discoverer of the X Ray*, pp. 100–101.

Chapter 3: X-rays in Medicine

18. Quoted in Nitske, *The Life of Wilhelm Conrad Röntgen, Discoverer of the X Ray*, p. 113.
19. Quoted in Penn State Milton S. Hershey Medical Center, Department of Radiology, "Edwards' XL Cathodal Plates." www.xray.hmc.psu.edu/rci/ss3/ss3_2.html.
20. Quoted in Nitske, *The Life of Wilhelm Conrad Röntgen, Discoverer of the X Ray*, p. 121.
21. Quoted in E.R.N. Grigg, *The Trail of the Invisible Light: From X-Strahlen to Radio(bio)logy*. Springfield, IL: Charles C. Thomas, 1965, p. 36.
22. Quoted in Nitske, *The Life of Wilhelm Conrad Röntgen, Discoverer of the X Ray*, p. 100.
23. Quoted in Glasser, *William Conrad Röntgen and the Early History of the Röntgen Rays*, p. 238.
24. Quoted in Nitske, *The Life of Wilhelm Conrad Röntgen, Discoverer of the X Ray*, pp. 115–16.
25. Quoted in John D. Bullock, letter to the editor, *Yale Medicine*, Summer 1998. http://info.med.yale.edu/external/pubs/ym_su98/letters/html.
26. Quoted in Grigg, *The Trail of the Invisible Light*, p. 30.
27. Quoted in Catherine Caulfield, *Multiple Exposures: Chronicles of the Radiation Age*. New York: Harper and Row, 1989, p. 10.
28. Quoted in Bettyann Holtzmann Kevles, *Naked to the Bone: Medical Imaging in the Twentieth Century*. New Brunswick, NJ: Rutgers University Press, 1997, p. 47.

29. Quoted in Joel D. Howell, *Technology in the Hospital: Transforming Patient Care in the Early Twentieth Century.* Baltimore: Johns Hopkins University Press, 1995, p. 108.

Chapter 4: Therapeutic Uses of X-rays

30. Quoted in Ronald L. Eisenberg, *Radiology: An Illustrated History.* St. Louis: Mosby-Year Book, 1992, p. 486.
31. Quoted in Eisenberg, *Radiology*, p. 481.
32. Quoted in Ruth Brecher and Edward Brecher, *The Rays: A History of Radiology in the United States and Canada.* Baltimore: Williams and Wilkins, 1969, p. 94.
33. Quoted in Brecher and Brecher, *The Rays*, p. 95.
34. Quoted in Brecher and Brecher, *The Rays*, p. 96.
35. Marie Curie, "The Discovery of Radium," address at Vassar College, May 14, 1921, reprinted in *Modern History Sourcebook*, Fordham University. www.fordham.edu/halsall/mod/curie-radium.html.

Chapter 5: Improving Medical Imaging

36. Quoted in Brecher and Brecher, *The Rays*, p. 33.
37. Quoted in Kevles, *Naked to the Bone*, p. 151.
38. Quoted in *Diagnostic Imaging Online*, "CT Inventor Godfrey Hounsfield Dies," August 19, 2004. www.dimag.com/dinews/2004081901.shtml.
39. Quoted in Kevles, *Naked to the Bone*, p. 167.
40. Jean P. Fisher, "Hospital Expansion System Is in Dispute," *Raleigh-Durham News and Observer*, July 28, 2004. www.newsobserver.com/business/story/1473227p-7618360c.html.
41. Brian Lentle, "The Magnetic Resonance Imperative," *Canadian Association of Radiologists Journal*, April 1999. http://collection.nlc-bnc.ca/100/201/300/cdn_medical_association/carj/vol-50/issue-2/0079.htm.

Chapter 6: Images of the Future

42. Quoted in Michele Meyer, "Behind the Body Scan Craze," *AARP Bulletin Online*, October 2002. www.aarp.org/bulletin/yourhealth/Articles/a2003-08-01-bodyscan.html.

43. Quoted in Meyer, "Behind the Body Scan Craze."
44. Quoted in MSNBC.com, "Study: Full-Body Scans Raise Cancer Risk," August 31, 2004. www.msnbc.msn.com/id/5868785.
45. Quoted in Penelope Patsuris, "The Future of Digital Imaging: Catching Disease Before It Catches Us," Forbes.com, May 3, 2004. www.forbes.com/infoimaging/2004/05/03/cx_pp_0503molecular_ii.html.
46. Quoted in Laura Lane, "Biomarker Imaging Magnifies Nuts and Bolts of Disease," *Molecular Imaging Outlook*, September 2004. www.dimag.com/molecularimagingoutlook/2004sep/index/shtml.
47. Quoted in Kathy Kincade, "Digital Technologies Push Images Beyond Today's Boundaries," *Diagnostic Imaging* special edition, July 2001. www.diagnosticimaging.com/specialedition/it.shtml
48. Quoted in Kincade, "Digital Technologies Push Images Beyond Today's Boundaries."
49. Quoted in Douglas Page, "Wireless PDAs May Prove Useful for Image Interpretation," *Diagnostic Imaging Magazine Online*, September 27, 2004. www.diagnosticimaging.com/pacsweb/showArticle.jhtml?articleID=47903497.

For Further Reading

Books

Dennis Brindell Fradin, *Medicine: Yesterday, Today, and Tomorrow.* Chicago: Childrens, 1988. The author traces the field of medicine from ancient times to the present day. While a bit dated, the book discusses the historical development of diagnostic instruments and humanity's never-ending battle with disease.

Kimberly Garcia, *Wilhelm Roentgen and the Discovery of X-rays.* Bear, DE: Mitchell Lane, 2003. This book discusses how a German scientist's accidental discovery changed forever the way we view our bodies and forged the new medical specialty of radiology.

Marylou Morano Kjelle, *Raymond Damadian and the Development of MRI.* Bear, DE: Mitchell Lane, 2003. The author relates the story of how medical researcher Raymond Damadian developed a new way of scanning the body to diagnose disease.

Carla Kellough McClafferty, *The Head Bone's Connected to the Neck Bone.* New York: Farrar, Straus & Giroux, 2001. A lively, illustrated look at the discovery of X-rays.

Barbara Moe, *The Revolution in Medical Imaging*. New York: Rosen, 2003. A basic overview of modern imaging techniques, including X-rays, CT and MRI scans, plus nuclear medicine and ultrasound.

Robert Mulcahy, *Medical Technology: Inventing the Instruments.* Minneapolis: Oliver, 1997. This work describes how X-rays, the stethoscope, the thermometer, and other medical instruments were developed.

Naomi Pasachoff, *Marie Curie and the Science of Radioactivity*. New York: Oxford University Press, 1996. The author presents the story of Marie Curie's life and work as the discoverer of radium.

Suzanne Zannos, *Godfrey Hounsfield and the Invention of CAT Scans*. Bear, DE: Mitchell Lane, 2003. This book takes a brief look at Röntgen's discovery of X-rays and then relates how Hounsfield used that technology to develop the CAT scanner.

Web Sites

American Institute of Physics. "Marie Curie and the Science of Radioactivity." (www.aip.org/history/curie/contents.htm). This online exhibit by the Center for the History of Physics is a complete biography of Curie, including photos, quotes, a reading list, and links.

How Stuff Works. "How X-Rays Work." (http://science.howstuffworks.com/x-ray.htm). A great site that explains the science of X-rays in easy-to-understand text. Includes diagrams and links to related sites as well as links to pages on "How MRI Works" and "How CT Scans Work."

The Nobel Prizes. "Wilhelm Conrad Röntgen—Biography." (http://nobelprize.org/physics/laureates/1901/rontgen-bio.html). This site provides a biography of every Nobel Prize-winner, including Röntgen, Curie, Cormack, and Hounsfield. In addition, many pages include the prizewinner's Nobel lecture, articles on their particular field, and links to other sites of interest.

Penn State Milton S. Hershey Medical Center, Department of Radiology. "A Century of Radiology." (www.xray.hmc.psu.edu/rci/centennial.html). Developed for the one-hundredth anniversary of the discovery of X-rays, this site is a chronological history of X-rays. It includes numerous historical photographs.

WORKS CONSULTED

Books

Ruth Brecher and Edward Brecher, *The Rays: A History of Radiology in the United States and Canada*. Baltimore: Williams and Wilkins, 1969. A thorough and informative, if now dated, volume that traces the history of radiology in North America.

Catherine Caulfield, *Multiple Exposures: Chronicles of the Radiation Age*. New York: Harper and Row, 1989. This book details the dangers encountered throughout the history of radiation science, from Röntgen's discovery of X-rays to Russia's Chernobyl disaster.

Ronald L. Eisenberg, *Radiology: An Illustrated History*. St. Louis: Mosby-Year Book, 1992. A profusely illustrated history of radiology, including sections on diagnostic, therapeutic, and nonmedical uses of X-rays.

Otto Glasser, *William Conrad Röntgen and the Early History of the Röntgen Rays*. Springfield, IL: Charles C. Thomas, 1934. The classic work on Röntgen and the development of his X-rays in physics and medicine.

Vivian Grey, *Roentgen's Revolution: The Discovery of the X Ray*. Boston: Little, Brown, 1973. A short biography of Wilhelm Conrad Röntgen.

E.R.N. Grigg, *The Trail of the Invisible Light: From X-Strahlen to Radio(bio)logy*. Springfield, IL: Charles C. Thomas, 1965. A massive, profusely illustrated book that chronicles the development of X-ray machines and the

Works Consulted

advances made in radiology from Röntgen's discovery through the first half of the twentieth century.

Joel D. Howell, *Technology in the Hospital: Transforming Patient Care in the Early Twentieth Century*. Baltimore: Johns Hopkins University Press, 1995. The author examines various early diagnostic methodologies and how they related, sometimes adversely, to patient care.

Bettyann Holtzmann Kevles, *Naked to the Bone: Medical Imaging in the Twentieth Century*. New Brunswick, NJ: Rutgers University Press, 1997. The author examines the entire field of medical imaging, from X-rays to MRI-assisted surgery.

W. Robert Nitske, *The Life of Wilhelm Conrad Röntgen, Discoverer of the X Ray*. Tucson: University of Arizona Press, 1971. A thorough examination of Röntgen's life and the impact his discovery had on him and the world.

Roy Porter, ed., *The Cambridge Illustrated History of Medicine*. Cambridge, UK: Cambridge University Press, 1996. This book traces the interrelation of disease, health, and medicine over two thousand years of history.

Stanley Joel Reiser, *Medicine and the Reign of Technology*. Cambridge, UK: Cambridge University Press, 1978. The author, a doctor and a professor, traces the history of medical innovations and techniques, such as the stethoscope and the thermometer, and discusses the growing supremacy of technology in medical diagnosis.

Periodical

Sneh Bhargava, "The Ethics of New Technology," *World Health*, May/June 1995.

Internet Sources

John D. Bullock, letter to the editor, *Yale Medicine*, Summer 1998. http://info.med.yale.edu/external/pubs/ym_su98/letters/html.

Center for the Study of Technology and Society, "Today in Technology History: February 22." www.tecsoc.org/pubs/history/2002/feb22.htm.

Marie Curie, "The Discovery of Radium," address at Vassar College, May 14, 1921, reprinted in *Modern History Sourcebook*, Fordham University. www.fordham.edu/halsall/mod/curie-radium.html

Diagnostic Imaging.com, "Radiologist Builds a Practice on Remote Reads." www.dimag.com/viewpoint/?articleID=47903402.

Diagnostic Imaging Online, "CT Inventor Godfrey Hounsfield Dies," August 19, 2004. www.dimag.com/dinews/2004081901.shtml.

Jean P. Fisher, "Hospital Expansion System Is in Dispute," *Raleigh-Durham News and Observer*, July 28, 2004. www.newsobserver.com/business/story/1473227p-7618360c.html.

Kathy Kincade, "Digital Technologies Push Images Beyond Today's Boundaries," *Diagnostic Imaging* special edition, July 2001. www.diagnosticimaging.com/specialedition/it.shtml.

Laura Lane, "Biomarker Imaging Magnifies Nuts and Bolts of Disease," *Molecular Imaging Outlook*, September 2004. www.dimag.com/molecularimagingoutlook/2004sep/index/shtml.

Brian Lentle, "The Magnetic Resonance Imperative," *Canadian Association of Radiologists Journal*, April 1999. http://collection.nlc-bnc.ca/100/201/300/cdn_medical_association/carj/vol-50/issue-2/0079.htm.

Medical Imaging.org, "Smart Technology: Aiding Diagnosis and Productivity." http://medicalimaging.org/future/technology.cfm.

Michele Meyer, "Behind the Body Scan Craze," *AARP Bulletin Online*, October 2002. www.aarp.org/bulletin/yourhealth/Articles/a2003-08-01-bodyscan.html.

MSNBC.com, "Study: Full-Body Scans Raise Cancer Risk," August 31, 2004. www.msnbc.msn.com/id/5868785.

National Cancer Institute, "NCI FACT SHEET: Nasopharyngeal Radium Irradiation (NRI)." www.nci.nih.

gov/newscenter/pressrelease/NRI/print?page=&keyword.

Douglas Page, "Wireless PDAs May Prove Useful for Image Interpretation," *Diagnostic Imaging Magazine Online*, September 27, 2004. www.diagnosticimaging.com/pacsweb/showArticle.jhtml?articleID=47903497.

Penelope Patsuris, "The Future of Digital Imaging: Catching Disease Before It Catches Us," Forbes.com, May 3, 2004. www.forbes.com/infoimaging/2004/05/03/cx_pp_0503molecular_ii.html.

Penn State Milton S. Hershey Medical Center, Department of Radiology, "Edwards' XL Cathodal Plates." www.xray.hmc.psu.edu/rci/ss3/ss3_2.html.

RadiologyInfo.org, "Cardiac MRI (MRI of the Heart, Great Vessel, and Adjacent Structures)." www.radiologyinfo.org/content/mr_cardiac.htm.

INDEX

actinography, 44
adoption, of new technologies, 47–48, 53, 54, 56, 84
afterloaders, 69
Allbutt, Thomas, 18
Alzheimer's disease, 91–92
American Roentgen Ray Society, 88
amputations, 50
angiograms, 52
anodes, 30, 35
antibiotics, 59
assassinations, 7–11
astronomy, 72–73
atoms, 35, 65
Auenbrugger von Auenbrugg, Leopold, 19
autopsies, 21–22

Babylon, ancient, 12–13
barium platinocyanide, 33, 34, 45
Beaumont, William, 23
Becquerel, Antoine-Henri, 63
Bhargava, Sneh, 88
biomarkers, 92
blood, circulation of, 14–15
bloodletting, 14
blood vessels, 52, 79
Boveri, Theodor, 38
Bracewell, Ronald, 72–73
brachytherapy, 68–70
brain, 52, 71
    imaging, 73
    tumors, 67
breast cancer, 61–62
bullet wounds, 8, 9–10, 23, 48
Butler, Prescott, 48

calcium tungstate, 45

Califano, Joseph, 83
cancer, 50–51
    treatment of, 60–62, 64–70
cathode rays, 30–31
cathodes, 30, 35
cathodography, 44
cells, 89
Celsius, Anders, 18
Celsius scale, 18
certificate-of-need (CON) laws, 83–84
cervical cancer, 69
Chang, Paul, 94
charge-coupled devices (CCDs), 92
chemotherapy, 90
children, radiation therapy and, 66
cobalt 60, 67, 69
Cole, Lewis, 52
Columbia University, 48
computed tomography scan (CT scan), 11
    full-body scanning, 86–89
    how it works, 77–79
    invention of, 76–77
    pros and cons of, 79–80
computers, 72, 95
    medical imaging and, 74, 75
contrast medium, 51–52, 73, 78–79, 90
Coolidge, William, 53
Cooper, Kenneth, 87–88
Cormack, Allan, 74–75, 76
costs, 67, 83–85, 88
Crookes, William, 29–30
Crookes tube, 29–30, 33, 34
Curie, Marie, 62–64
Curie, Pierre, 63
Czolgosz, Leon, 7

Dally, Clarence, 47, 50
Dam, H. J. W., 32

INDEX

Damadian, Raymond, 82
Dandy, Walter, 52
darkrooms, 37–38
Dartmouth College, 47
data transmission, 94–95, 96
demons, 13
dermatitis, 49
diagnosis, 35, 41, 47–48, 52, 54
  body temperature and, 15–18
  future of, 97
  history of, 12–15
  medical imaging and, 79–80, 83, 87–88, 90
  PACS and, 94
diagraphy, 44
digestion, 23
dosimeters, 51

Edison, Thomas, 8, 45–46, 47, 71
Electrical Engineer (journal), 46
electrography, 44
electromagnetic spectrum, 58
electromagnets, 81
electrons, 30, 35
electroskiagraphy, 44
EMI, Limited, 75, 77
encephalograms, 52
endoscopes, 24
epilepsy, 12–13
ethics, medical, 88
Experiments and Observations on the Gastric Juice and the Physiology of Digestion (Beaumont), 23
eye diseases, 22

fads, 41–45, 53, 71
Fahrenheit, Daniel Gabriel, 17
Fahrenheit scale, 17–18
false positives, risk of, 88–89
Finsen, Neils, 58–59
Fisher, Jean P., 84
fluorography, 44
fluoroscopes, 45–47
Frankfurter Zeitung (newspaper), 41
Frost, Edwin B., 47–48
Frost, Gilman, 48

Galileo Galilei, 16
Gamma Knife, 67
gamma rays, 66, 72, 74, 76, 90
George Washington Medical Center, 9
germicides, 57–58

Greece, ancient, 13
Groote Schuur Hospital, 74
Grubbé, Emil, 61–62
gymnasiums (high schools), 27

hair loss, 49
Harvey, William, 14–15
health benefits
  of light, 57–59
  of MRI, 82
  see also treatment
health risks, 47, 48–51, 57, 62
  CT scan, 79–80
  full–body scanning, 88–89
  MRI, 82–83
  radiation, 64, 66
  surgery, 67, 68
hearing, sense of, 18–21
Hearst, William Randolph, 71
heart disease, 81
Helmholtz, Hermann von, 22
Hinkley, John, Jr., 8
Hippocrates, 13–14, 19
Historical Röntgen Committee (Chicago), 48
Hooke, Robert, 17
hospitals, 53, 83–84, 93–94, 96–97
hot cathode tube, 53
Hounsfield, Godfrey, 75–77, 90
humors, theory of, 13–14

imaging centers, 97
Internet, the, 94–95, 97
Internet2, 94–95
Ishaque, Nadeem, 91
ixography, 44

Johns Hopkins Hospital, 52
Jones, Philip Mills, 59

Kevles, Bettyann Holtzmann, 72
Kieffer, Jean, 55, 77
Kodak Health Imaging, 95

Laënnec, René-Théophile-Hyacinthe, 19–21
laws, 43, 83–84
lead, 35, 38, 51
Lee, Rose, 62
Leeuwenhoek, Antoni van, 17
Lenard, Philipp, 33, 40
Lentle, Brian, 84–85
Life of Wilhelm Conrad Röntgen,

Discoverer of the X Ray, The, (Nitske), 32, 40, 44
linear accelerators, 65–67
lupus vulgaris, 59

magnetic resonance imaging (MRI), 11, 80–83, 97
magnets, 30, 81
Martin, M. F., 43
Massachusetts Institute of Technology, 49
McCarthy, Eddie, 48
McKinley, William, 7–8, 10–11
medical imaging
  costs of, 83–85
  future of, 97
  history of, 24–25
  pioneers of, 72–75
  see also specific imaging techniques
MedicalImaging.org, 95
medical schools, 47, 49
mercury, 18
metals, 35
microscopes, 17
microwaves, 66
military use, 53–54
mobile units, 54
modesty, 43

Naked to the Bone: Medical Imaging in the Twentieth Century (Kevles), 72
nasopharyngeal radium irradiation (NRI), 66
Nation (magazine), 47
neutrons, 35
New Jersey legislature, 43
"New Kind of Rays, A" (Wilhelm Röntgen), 39, 40
newspapers, 41–43, 49
New World Journal (newspaper), 71
nighthawks, 96–97
Nitske, W. Robert, 32, 40, 44
Nobel Prize
  for Chemistry, 64
  for Medicine, 59, 75, 77
  for Physics, 40, 64
Northwestern University, 96

obsessions, scientific, 32
Oldendorf, William, 72, 73
On Mediate Auscultation (Laënnec), 21
opera glasses, 43

ophthalmology, 22
ophthalmoscopes, 22–24
oranges, 73–74

Pan American Exposition, 7
Parr, Jerry, 8, 9
particle accelerators, 65
patents, 44–45, 74
pellets, radioactive, 69
personal digital assistants (PDAs), 95–96
Phelps, Michael, 92
Philadelphia Medical Journal, 60
photographic plates, 36–37, 43, 53
photography, 24–25, 28, 43, 92
physicians, 47–48, 54, 56
  medical imaging and, 84–85
Physico–Medical Society (Würtzburg), 39
physics, 28, 29–30, 65
picture archive and communication systems (PACS), 93–94
pilots, radiation therapy and, 66
pneumoencephalography, 73
polonium, 64
popular culture, 86
portraits, 44
positron emission tomography (PET), 11, 89–90, 92
preventive health care, 88
prostate cancer, 69
protective clothing, 51
protons, 35
publication, of scientific discoveries, 39, 74, 82
Pupin, Michael, 48
pyknoscopy, 44

radiation
  cancer treatment and, 60–62, 64–70
  Marie Curie and, 63–64
  measurement of, 51
  radioactive solutions and, 90
  risks of, 48–52, 79–80, 88–89
radio frequency waves, 82
radiologists, 49, 96–97
radiology. *See* medical imaging; X-rays
RadiologyInfo.org, 81
radiometer, 29
radiotelescopes, 73
radiotherapy
  external, 65–68
  internal, 68–70
radium, 62, 64, 66

Index

Reagan, Ronald, 8–11
Reiser, Stanley Joel, 18–19, 21
remote medicine, 94–97
Röentgen Rays in Medicine and Surgery, The (Williams), 49
roentgens, 51
Röntgen, Bertha, 26, 38–39
Röntgen, Charlotte, 26
Röntgen, Friedrich, 26
Röntgen, Wilhelm
   cathode ray experiments and, 30–33
   discovery by, 33–39, 40
   patents of, 44–45
   youth and education of, 26–28
Röntgen rays, 44, 45
Roosevelt, Theodore, 7
Ruhmkorff coils, 31, 33, 34, 43

Santorio, Santorio, 16
scanners, text, 75
science fiction, 86
scuba divers, radiation therapy and, 66
seeds, radioactive, 69
sight, sense of, 21–24
skin conditions, 49, 58–60, 61
Skinner, Clarence E., 61
"Smart Technology: Aiding Diagnosis and Productivity" (article), 95
snow, measurement of, 75
soft tissues, 51–52
souvenirs, 44
Stanley, Robert J., 88–89
Stenbeck, Thor, 61
stereotactic radiosurgery, 67
stereotactic radiotherapy, 68
stethoscopes, 20–21
St. Martin, Alexis, 23
submarine crews, radiation therapy and, 66
sunlight, 57
Superman, 86
surgery, 21, 48, 65, 67, 83
Swiss Avalanche Center, 75

telemedicine, 96–97
teleradiology, 96–97
temperature, diagnosing disease and, 15–18
thallium, 29
thermometers, 16–18
thermoscopes, 16–17

tithonography, 44
tomography, 55–56, 75
   see also computed tomography scan
touch, sense of, 19
treatment
   in ancient times, 13, 14
   of bullet wounds, 8, 9–10, 23, 48
   of cancer, 60–62, 64–70
   of skin conditions, 57–60
tuberculosis, 52
Tufts University, 74

ultraviolet (UV) light, 58–59
University of Giessen, 28
University of Strasbourg, 28
University of Würzburg, 28
uranium, 63–64
U.S. Army Medical Corps., 54
Utrecht University, 27

vacuum tubes, 29–30, 32, 35, 60–61
videoconferencing, 96

Waitz, Aaron, 95
Williams, Francis Henry, 49
wireless technology, 95
World Health (journal), 88
World War I, 54

X-ray detectors, 77
X-rays
   acceptance of, 47–48, 53, 54, 56
   advancements in, 51–53
   digital, 92–93
   discovery of, 33–39, 40
   future of, 95
   health risks of, 47, 48–51, 57, 62
   how they work, 35
   names for, 44
   nonmedical uses of, 43–44, 56
   remote interpretation of, 96–97
X-ray studios, 43–44, 53
X-ray technicians, 51, 94
X-ray tubes, 77

Yaghmai, Yahid, 96

Picture Credits

Cover: © Jose Luis Pelaez, Inc./CORBIS
AP Wide World Photos, 31, 87
© Araldo de Luca/CORBIS
Bernd Weissbrod/DPA/Landov, 84
© Bettmann/CORBIS, 9, 23, 46
© Dr. Robert Friedland/Photo Researchers, Inc., 91
© Hulton Archive/Getty Images, 29, 76
© Hulton-Deutsch Collection/CORBIS, 50, 63
Jens Wolf/DPA/Landov, 93
© Lester Lefkowitz/CORBIS, 10
Marianne DuPlain, 36, 58, 78
© Roger Ressmeyer/CORBIS, 68, 70
© Science Photo Library/Photo Researchers, Inc., 53
© Simon Fraser/Royal Victoria Infirmary, Newcastle Upon Tyne/Photo Researchers, Inc., 81
© Swim Ink 2, LLC/CORBIS, 42
U.S. National Library of Medicine, 15, 17, 20, 27, 37, 55, 72
© Volker Steger/Photo Researchers, Inc., 80, 96

About the Author

Craig E. Blohm has written magazine articles on historical subjects for children for the past twenty years, and he has authored several books for Lucent Books. He has written for social studies textbooks and conducted workshops in writing history for children. A native of Chicago, Blohm and his wife, Desiree, live in Tinley Park, Illinois, and have two sons, Eric and Jason.